THE SHOCKING TRUTH OF PARACETAMOL

A HANDBOOK FOR EFFECTIVE MANAGEMENT OF FEVER AND FLU WITHOUT DRUGS

Dr. Kamalpreet Singh

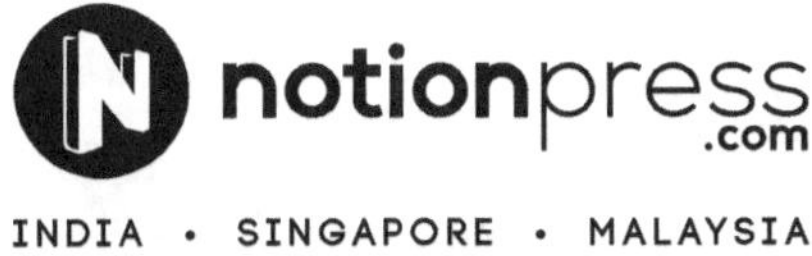

INDIA • SINGAPORE • MALAYSIA

ISBN 979-8-88909-891-1

My Sincere Gratitude to The Almighty

for blessing me with

Strength, Courage, and Perseverance

to walk the path of

Truth, Freedom, and Health.

DISCLAIMER

The text, graphics, images, and other material contained in this book are for informational purposes only. No material in this book is intended to be a substitute for professional medical advice, diagnosis, or treatment. Always seek the advice of your physician or other qualified health care provider with any questions you may have regarding a medical condition or treatment and before undertaking a new health care regimen, and never disregard professional medical advice or delay in seeking it because of something you have read in this book.

ABOUT THE AUTHOR

Dr. Kamalpreet Singh is a leading diabetes reversal specialist, clinical researcher, and medical nutritionist with over five years of experience in type-2 diabetes remission. He has successfully assisted more than 100 individuals to reverse diabetes through evidence-based nutrition and metabolic health strategies.

Dr. Singh serves as a Clinical Researcher at the Hospital and Institute of Integrated Medical Sciences (HIIMS), where he pioneers plant-based disease reversal protocols and integrative nutrition therapies. His expertise is backed by multiple international certifications, including Plant-Based Nutrition from Cornell University, Diabetes Reversal Coaching from the Institute of Food and Nutrition Therapy, and Fitness Nutrition from the American Council on Exercise.

Recognized for his outstanding contributions to plant-based disease reversal, he is a Dietitian under the Indo-Vietnam Medical Board and an honorary doctorate recipient for his groundbreaking contributions to medical nutrition. He is a member of esteemed medical networks, including the Network of Influenza Care Experts and Wellness & Inflammatory Syndrome Experts.

Dr. Singh has authored eight peer-reviewed research articles on diabetes reversal in leading medical journals, including the International Journal of Disease Reversal and Prevention, the Journal of Science of Healing Outcomes, and Ayushdhara Academic Journal. He has also been awarded by the India Book of Records for an extraordinary track record in medical nutrition services. A prolific author, he has written five books, including Advanced Nutrition Therapy, P.O.S.H. Way to Reverse Type-2 Diabetes, and The Vaccine Crime Report. His insights into holistic healing have made him a sought-after lecturer and keynote speaker at international health conferences, medical seminars, and wellness workshops.

Dr. Singh is also an expert in fasting and detoxification, having personally undertaken extended fasting protocols, such as 40-day grain fasting, 30-day juice fasting, 18-day coconut water fasting, and 9-day water fasting. His deep personal experience in fasting and detoxification has further shaped his innovative approach to healing.

As the innovator of the Supervised Diabetes Reversal Coaching Program, he integrates Moderate Glycemic Load diet strategies and Insulin Sensitivity Optimization techniques to help individuals restore their metabolic health naturally. His insights have been featured in international media, where he continues to advocate for a nutrition-first approach to healthcare.

Through his groundbreaking research, clinical expertise, and writing, Dr. Kamalpreet Singh is on a mission to redefine the future of healthcare—where food is the key to healing, prevention is the priority, and chronic diseases are no longer a life sentence.

FOLLOW THE AUTHOR

Dr. Kamalpreet Singh
WhatsApp: +1 416 795 1002
Website: https://gosatvik.ca/
Email: kamalpreetsingh@gosatvik.ca
Telegram: https://t.me/gosatvik
Twitter: https://twitter.com/gosatvik
Instagram: https://www.instagram.com/gosatvik
YouTube: https://www.youtube.com/@drksinghkhalsa

CONTENTS

Wherever there is a problem, there is an underlying cause of the problem. The solution to the problem is to remove the cause of the problem. To remove the cause of the problem, we need to identify and understand the cause. Isn't it?

If you are suffering from any health problem, and you go to a medical doctor, all you might get to hear is to get yourself tested, take a drug, pop some pills, maybe remove your organs, or replace them with someone else's organs and this is the only solution offered to you for every health problem. As you trust the doctor, you might also believe the story that these are the only options left for you. You might be holding a belief that the doctor would understand your disease and its cure as he spent long years in the medical school. Therefore, what he tells should be correct as a rule of thumb. Unfortunately, you do not realise that <u>the syllabus of the medical schools is designed to profit the pharmaceutical companies at the cost of your health.</u>

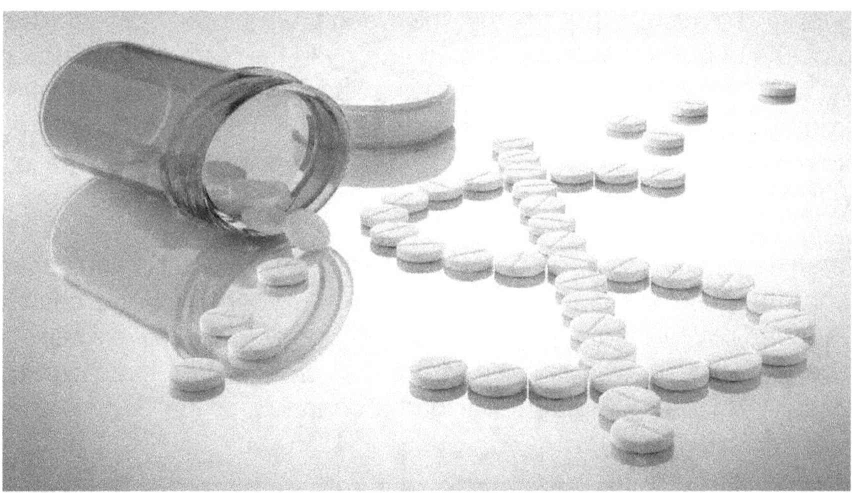

So, you take his advice and pop some pills that suppress the symptoms of your disease, and you start feeling better. However, the relief does not last long. Every time you stop taking the drugs, the problem reappears, and it is much worse than it was before.

This is because the drugs do not remove the root cause of the problem. They are not designed to remove the cause but only suppress the symptoms. With the passage of time, the side effects of the drugs add up with the cause of the initial disease, until it comes to a point when it's too late to do anything.

To treat an illness associated with an organ, it is critical to understand how a cell in an organ dies. It will help you understand the reason for your illness and suffering. It will give you hope that your illness can be reversed, and you can restore health. Have you wondered, what is the cause of all these diseases?

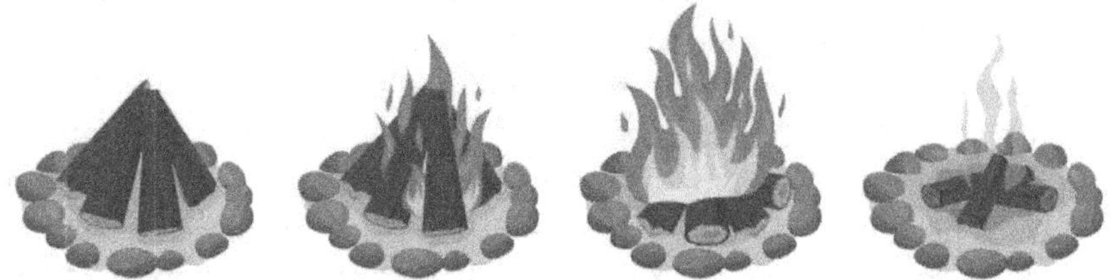

Let me explain in a simple manner. Let us take an example of a bonfire. The woods to be placed in the bonfire have some stored energy. To access that energy, the woods need to be burned. The process of burning would produce energy in the form of heat along with some waste in the form of ashes. These ashes are the residue (remains) of the process. A similar process can be observed in the human body. In the process, the body also produces ashes or wastes.

Imagine you picked up an orange and started eating it. Do you know what happens to the orange when it leaves your hand and enters your body? Well, that orange passes through your digestive system. The body keeps what it needs from that orange, and the residual waste is excreted through four detox channels of the body in the form of SUBS:

Stool	To throw the wastes from the intestines
Urine	To throw the wastes from the kidneys
Breathe	To throw the wastes from the lungs
Sweat	To throw the wastes from the skin

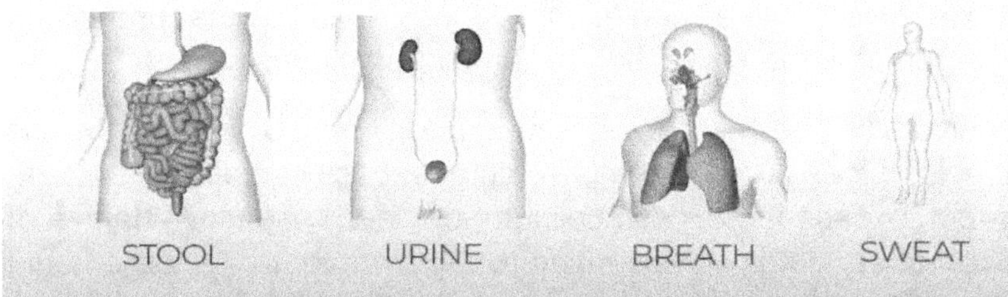

Now, because of our wrong food choices, wrong lifestyle, and environmental factors, our body and vitality undergo enervation. As a result, some of the detox channels are not able to work as efficiently as required to ensure smooth functioning of the body. As a result, the waste matter starts accumulating in the body. Accumulation of the toxic waste is the major cause of most chronic diseases[1].

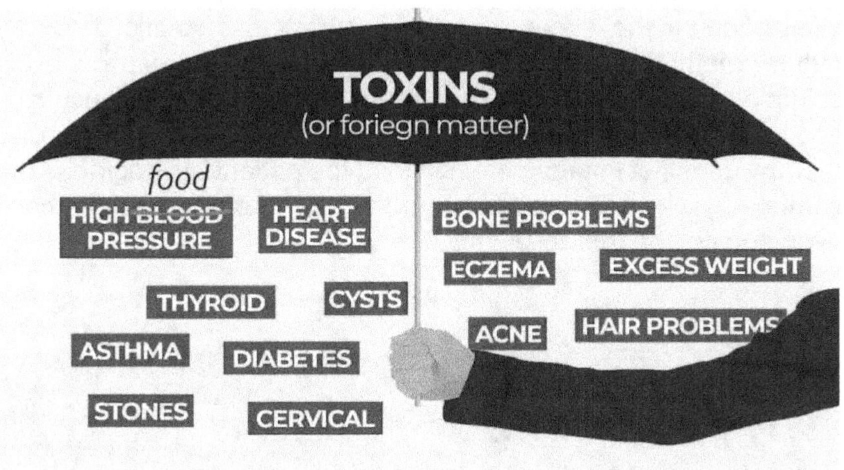

You are told that you have diabetes, hypertension, kidney failure, fatty liver, obesity, eczema, etc. but try to understand that these are different names given by the medical industry to the variety of symptoms that appear due to the accumulated toxic waste in various parts of the body. The waste can be stored near the brain, heart, lungs, etc. causing organ specific diseases. If the waste is stored near the blood vessels of the heart, then the disease will cause suffering to the cardiac cells. Similarly, if the waste is stored near the kidney, then the kidney cells will not have adequate access to oxygen and the cells will start dying. This will result in kidney disease or in critical conditions, kidney failure. The underlying cause remains the same, i.e., accumulation of wastes.

This waste can be called excess mucous, excess creatinine, excess uric acid, excess urea, excess sodium, excess cholesterol, excess bilirubin, excess fat, excess calcium, etc. and respective names of the diseases are given according to the symptoms. As the amount of waste being produced and stored in the body is more than the amount of waste being eliminated, over a period of time, all the organs get affected by disease due to the interconnectedness of the human body. Therefore, the mechanism of getting sick is the inability of the body to eliminate excess waste[2]. So, we have identified the cause of the problem now.

The real solution of any problem lies in eradicating the cause of the problem. Similarly, the cure of modern chronic diseases lies in the elimination of the excess waste through a systematic detox by natural methods. People think that big problems would need big solutions, and in this belief, they even agree to undergo most toxic and deadly treatments and therapies like chemotherapy[3]. This toxic therapy does not improve the health of the patient but degrades the immune system to such an extent that some of the patients can't even survive the therapy itself.

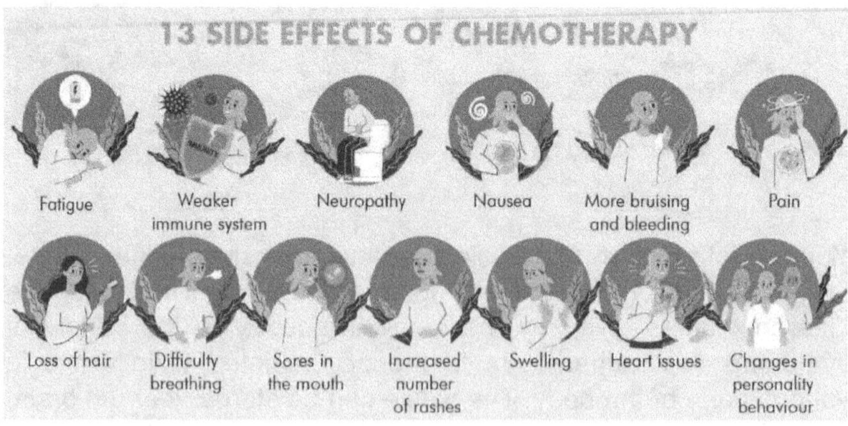

We must understand that the solution may not need ultra-scientific approach towards a disease but just common sense, which most of the modern-day medical doctors lack. Let us understand this with the help of an analogy.

Imagine that you are a caretaker of an aquarium. You love and take care of the fish inside. Despite of all your care, the water in the aquarium gets polluted after a period of time. As a result, a fish falls sick. Now think yourself what you would do if you or a member of your family fell sick. You would visit the doctor! So, you decided to take the sick fish to a medical doctor.

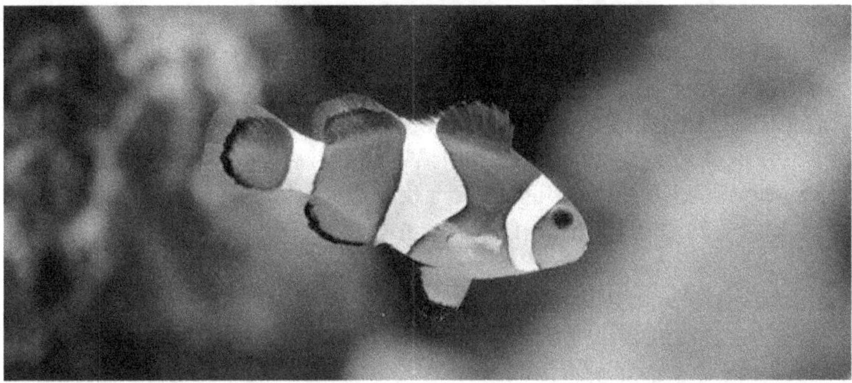

The doctor upon examining the fish gave some tablets and told that the fish must take it for a week and will be cured from the disease. You became happy when the fish started recovering. Since the water was still polluted, after some days the fish fell sick again. This time, the symptoms were a little more serious. You did not want to take any risk. So, you decided to take the fish to the best hospital of the city. The doctor advised you to admit the fish in the hospital for a few days. Some injections and medication did the magic again. The fish recovered and got discharged from the hospital. You again dropped the fish into its house, i.e., aquarium. But again, after a few days the fish got seriously ill. This time the general physician referred him to a specialist and upon testing, the specialist doctor revealed that the fish is diabetic and must take metformin (diabetes pill) two times a day for the rest of its life and everything will be perfect. You trained the fish to follow the doctor's advice religiously. Despite all the best efforts from fish and you, after some time the fish fell sick again!

So, the question is "what is the cause of the sickness"? What do you do now? Where is the problem? By now you must have understood the moral of the story. The problem was never in the fish! It was the polluted water! You simply must change the water. Even the best doctor of the world will not be able to cure the fish if it continues to live in the polluted water. Trying to cure the fish without changing the water is like chasing a mirage. Every time it will appear that the cure is nearby, but you will never be able to achieve it. In this process, you will drain your health and wealth.

For example, diabetes type-2 is not a disease in which you require the knowledge of advanced microbiology to understand the problem. It is just a specific homeostatic condition of the body which can be understood and corrected with a reform in diet and lifestyle[4]. I have helped 100s of people reverse type-2 diabetes by switching to a whole-food plant-based diet. Within few weeks of switching to my suggested diet and lifestyle plan, the blood glucose readings start stabilizing and within a few months, my clients are able to maintain normal blood sugar readings without taking any medication like metformin. You can read about this process of natural healing in my book 'Advanced Nutrition Therapy: Goodbye Drugs and Diseases.'

Now, since the subject of this book is to educate you in the effective management of fever and other related symptoms, let us try to understand, why do we get fevers, colds, coughs, diarrhea, etc. and should we fear them? Are they harmful? Should we suppress them with drugs like paracetamol (popularly known by the brand name "Tylenol")? What are the direct and long-term side effects of using such drugs? Are flu shots safe and effective? If we do not take any chemical-based drugs, then what is the natural and safe way to manage fever effectively? Let us find out.

A cold, cough, or fever should not be feared but celebrated. It seems illogical, doesn't it? Let me explain that cold, cough, fever, diarrhea, vomiting, etc. these are called first stage diseases and they last for a short time. They're actually an attempt by our immune system to get rid of the toxic overload that has been accumulating inside our body over the past months and years. These are not really illnesses but the symptoms of a process which attempts to keep you healthy. I like to call them happy diseases.

Just like we clean our house every day, but once or twice a year, we carry out a much more thorough "Master Cleanse" when we lift all the rugs, sofas, bed, etc. and sweep below them too. In the same way once or twice every year, even our body carries out much more thorough "Master Cleanse" through cold, coughs, vomiting, diarrhea, and these are called first stage diseases.

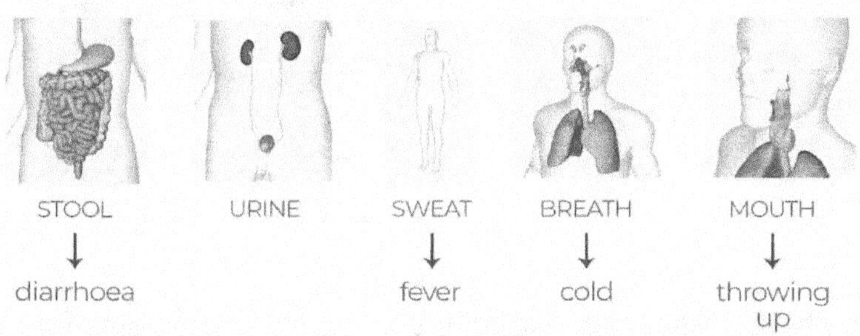

You must remember that we have four channels of detox in our body through which waste matter passes out in the form of Stool, Urine, Breath and Sweat (SUBS) which eliminate toxic wastes from the body. During happy diseases, the effectiveness of one of the four detox channels is increased or a fifth channel is opened. For example, during a fever the effectiveness of our sweat channel increases, during diarrhea the effectiveness of our stool channel increases, during common cold the effectiveness of our nose channel increases and when we throw up, a fifth channel to eliminate the excess of toxins is opened.

Unfortunately, the first thing that you do when you develop a cold is run to a medical doctor and ask the doctor to give you something that stops your runny nose. Do you see the problem? What you're basically saying is, "Hey, give me something that stops these toxins from escaping my body!" You take the drug, it manipulates and interferes with your immune system, and the cold stops because the toxins that your body was trying to throw out are pushed back inside. Drugs do not cure; they suppress the disease. That is why I do not call them medicines. People have been so brainwashed by pharmaceutical companies and medical doctors that it's difficult to make them understand that these things are the body's attempt to heal itself.

If natural drugless methods are adopted during such acute disease (like cold, coughs, fevers, etc.) and if no attempt is made to suppress it through any drugs, the further two stages of disease to be described would never be there[5]. Now what happens when you repeatedly keep suppressing these toxins inside?

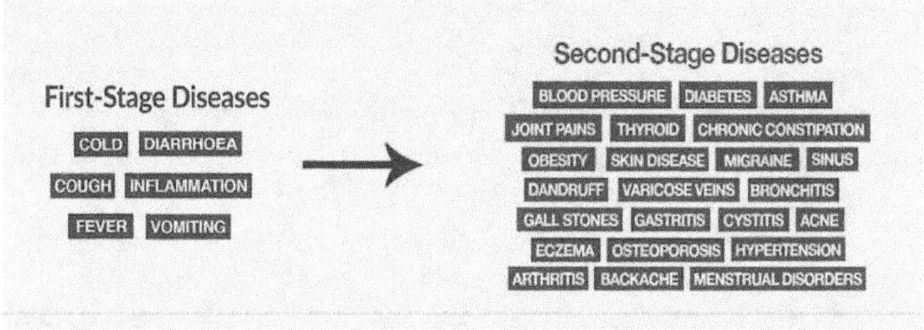

These happy diseases take their second stage that lasts for longer periods of time such as hypertension, diabetes, asthma, thyroid, constipation, obesity, migraines, varicose veins, bronchitis, gall stones, gastritis, cystitis, acne, eczema, arthritis, backache, menstrual disorders, etc. Can you guess what happens when you further suppress second-stage diseases inside your body by drugs?

They take the third stage that are destructive like heart attacks, cancers, kidney failure, strokes, brain tumors, Parkinson's disease, etc. You know you have a third stage disease when death could be near at hand.

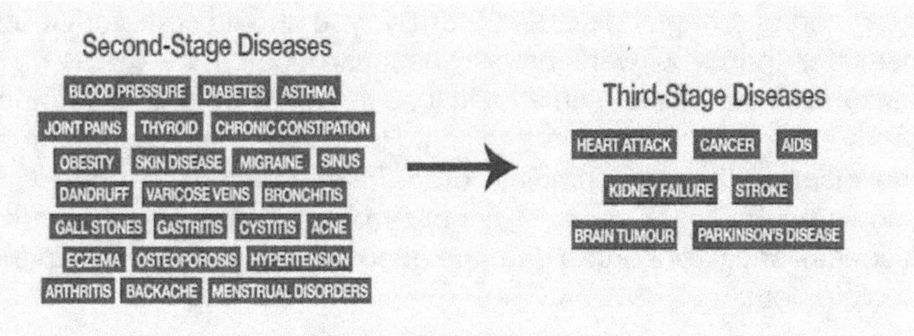

Let not the acute disease be suppressed. No chronic disease can develop in the person[1]. However, the good news is that at any of these three stages you can very well take a U-turn, correct your mistakes, reform your lifestyle, and begin a new journey towards a healthy and disease-free life.

Society often conditions us to think that these illnesses are something bad, something unpleasant, something to be fought against. But it's quite the opposite. Colds, fevers, vomiting, diarrhea - these illnesses come to detoxify and clean our body. They are an attempt by the immune system to get rid of all that waste, the toxins lying inside. When we eat unnatural, refined, and processed foods like pasta, noodles, biscuits, ice creams, sugar, it does not get digested properly and accumulates inside the body as toxic matter. Besides that, when we consume or inject anything made with chemicals, it is foreign to the human body and thus requires elimination. When these aren't eliminated properly, it gets stored as toxins and give rise to various diseases.

But our immune system is very powerfully designed. Once or twice a year, it opens one of these four detox channels so that the undigested accumulated waste can get out. So, if you have colds, coughs, fevers, diarrhea, etc. instead of viewing it as something unpleasant you should be grateful that you have got a chance to detoxify your body. When you take a drug to suppress your symptoms, the waste that your immune system was so desperately trying to throw out is pushed back in. If you keep resorting to these 'quick fixes', soon you'll have a bigger problem, and it would require much more time to heal.

After curing a happy disease naturally, you should come out much healthier than you were before, because your body would have thrown out the waste. You should lose the extra weight, have much more energy and clarity in thinking. However, when you suppress the disease through chemical drugs like Paracetamol, popularly known by the brand name 'Tylenol', you are inviting much chronic diseases and latent organ damage about which you will study in this book in detail.

It is because most people are not aware of the fact that fever is not an illness itself. Fever is defined as an increase in the normal set point of body temperature[6]. Acute childhood illnesses are often associated with fever, which is considered by parents and by many doctors as a major and harmful sign of illness, sometimes as an illness itself rather than a symptom of a host defense response. Fever is normal part of the body response to fight the infection; the body temperature is well controlled in the brain and does not rise relentlessly. The accumulated data suggests that fever has a protective role in promoting host defense against infection. A moderate fever (less than 40°C) is beneficial[7]. There is no evidence that fever itself worsens the course of an illness or that it causes long-term neurologic complications[8]. Fever is rarely harmful and only extremely high fevers of 42.2°C (108°F) may cause brain damage. However, fevers of 41°C (106°F) should get immediate medical attention to examine the patient for severe infection according to an article published in BMC Pediatrics[6].

When we focus upon 'treating' the fever, we are giving the impression to parents and health professionals that fever is harmful and that antipyresis is beneficial. Scientific evidence does not support this practice. To continue the current practice of liberal use of antipyretics may mean that we are ignoring important messages from research[7].

Current Practise amongst Pediatricians and Parents

Majority of the parents have a poor understanding of fever and its beneficial role in diseases[9]. An exaggerated fear of fever, called fever phobia, is common among parents. They worry when their child is feverish and feel that fever may spiral upwards with a possible fatal outcome. As a result, they are convinced that antipyretic measures must be used to lower fever[10]. Many parents administer antipyretics like paracetamol, even when there is minimal fever because they are concerned that their child must maintain a "normal" temperature[8]. The blockage of fever with antipyretics interferes with normal immunological development in the brain and may lead to neurodevelopmental disorders[6].

Parents do not realise that they are constructing a path of suffering and illness for themselves as well as their children. How can they be aware? Who will spread the awareness? The pharmaceutical companies? Of course not! Well, if they educate the people that fever is not an illness itself; it should not be feared; it is a beneficial mechanism of self-cleansing; and it should not be suppressed with drugs; then how would they sell the drugs like paracetamol and dozens of its brand names? How will they generate the billion-dollar sales revenue? Who will get the side effects that fetch them lifelong customers for chronic illnesses?

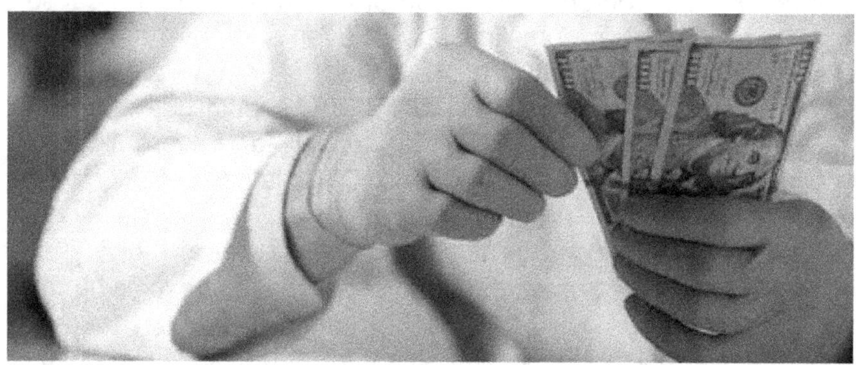

Will medical doctors educate the people? Why not? The truth is that the majority of medical doctors themselves aren't fully aware of fever and its beneficial role. There is often a wide perception among pediatricians that fever is dangerous. Although most pediatricians agree that treatment of a febrile child with antipyretics is mostly for the relief of the symptoms of fever, many tend to prescribe antipyretics for any child with fever. Pediatricians contribute to fever phobia by prescribing antipyretics for children who are only mildly febrile or by recommending the use of paracetamol alternating with ibuprofen[7]. Acetaminophen and ibuprofen are commonly used in an alternating manner for management of fever. There is presently no scientific evidence that this combination is safe or achieves faster antipyresis than either agent alone. There is evidence that the improper use of these agents may cause harm[11]. There are a few doctors who do their diligent research, study the evidence, and gather the courage to stand up and point out that drug-based intensive treatment is a health hazard which should not be neglected. These honest doctors are quickly silenced by the authorities. They are discredited, scorned, and their work is not published. They have to face a lot of heat from their peers and medical boards. I respect and support them from the bottom of my heart.

Fever by itself is self-limiting and rarely serious provided that the cause is known, and fluid loss is replaced. With fever, unlike hyperthermia, body temperature is well regulated by a hypothalamic set-point that balances heat production and heat loss so effectively that the temperature does not climb up relentlessly and does not exceed an upper limit of 42°C. Within this upper range, 40°C to 42°C, there is no evidence that the fever is injurious to tissue. About 20% of children seen in the emergency room have temperatures over 40°C but they usually have a full recovery. If there is morbidity or mortality, it is due to the underlying disease. The associated fever may well be protective[7]. The following are some benefits of fever as described in the medical literature:

- Fever exerts an overall adverse effect on the growth of bacteria and on replication of viruses[12-13]. It also enhances immunological processes, including activity of interleukin-1 (IL-1), T-helper cells, cytolytic T-cells, B-cell, and immunoglobulin synthesis[7]. IL-1 is more active at febrile temperature than at an afebrile temperature. Interferon (INF), a potent antiviral agent, has enhanced antiviral activity above 40°C[7].

- The mobility, phagocytosis and killing of bacteria by polymorphonuclear leukocytes are significantly greater at temperatures above 40°C. Elevated temperatures of 38°C and 39°C have a direct positive effect on lymphocyte transformation, the generation of cytolytic cells, B-cell activity, and immunoglobulin synthesis[14].

- A study of about one hundred children with salmonella gastroenteritis from Finland demonstrated a significant negative correlation between the degree of fever and the duration of excretion of organisms[15].

- In a series of children presenting with severe infections, such as pneumonia or septicemia, it was found that the lower the body temperature, the higher the mortality[16].

➤ Insufflations of humidified air at 43°C (3 sessions of 30 minutes at intervals of 3 hours) into the nasal passages of patients suffering from coryza resulted in the suppression of symptoms in 78% of the patients[17].

➤ In human volunteers infected with rhinovirus, the use of antipyretics was associated with suppression of serum antibody response, increased symptoms and signs and a trend towards longer duration of viral shedding[18].

➤ Early exposure to infections and fevers protects children from developing allergic diseases according to the hygiene theory[19]. Fever is metabolically expensive: every 1°C rise in temperature increases the metabolic rate by approximately 10%[6].

➤ The use of antipyretics to suppress fever results in an increased mortality rate in bacterially infected rabbits[20]. The use of antipyretics to suppress fever increases influenza virus production in ferrets[21].

➤ Fever enhances the immune response by increasing mobility and activity of white cells[22-24]. Fever has been associated with a decreased morbidity and mortality rate in a variety of infections[25-26]. A meta-analysis conducted in 2016-17 reveals that a person who has fever while being infected has a lesser chance of dying[27].

In light of the findings of the above scientific studies, we can conclude that we do not need to fear a fever but allow it to run its course to support our life in various ways. Fever itself is not an illness. However, when a person gets a fever, there is an associated discomfort with it. You might think, "Oh! If fever is beneficial, then why do I feel excessive weakness and fatigue? Why am I not able to enjoy my fever day as a normal day, playing and enjoying? Why am I experiencing pain all over my body. Also, why have I lost taste and hunger? What about the diarrhea, cough and cold?"

First, let us understand why happy diseases cause us discomfort. As we have discussed, because of our wrong food choices, wrong lifestyle, and environmental factors, our body and vitality undergo enervation. As a result, some of the detox channels are not able to work as efficiently as required to ensure smooth functioning of the body. As a result, the waste matter starts accumulating in the body. Accumulation of the toxic waste is the major cause of most chronic diseases[1].

Now, the body does not want to remain full of wastes and toxins. It has an immune system, an in-built mechanism of self-healing. How long can the body tolerate the toxic conditions? Not indefinitely! When the waste (phlegm, mucus, etc.) have accumulated beyond the tolerance limit, the self-healing power asserts itself and instructs the body internally (as a signal) to stop following the disease-causing wrong diet and lifestyle. Once or twice a year, when that tolerance limit is reached, the immune system declares a condition of emergency within.

When such an emergency is declared, all the energy that would ordinarily be made available to the skeletal muscles for doing the everyday activities, carry out intellectual and physical functions like digestion of food, working daily jobs, etc. is withdrawn to a great extent and diverted to the concerned internal organs to vigorously eliminate waste matter in the form of cough, cold, fever, diarrhea, skin eruption, etc. This leads to a feeling of weakness, fatigue, body pains, loss of taste and hunger, etc. as the body wants you to avoid eating food and ensure complete rest for proper elimination of wastes.[5]

So, we have understood the reason for discomfort during happy diseases. Now, we will discuss the potential side effects of suppressing the happy diseases with antipyretics like paracetamol and then we would provide you an all-natural method of supporting your body through happy diseases.

PARACETAMOL ASSOCIATED RISKS

A growing body of evidence in the last decade suggests that the use of paracetamol blocks the body's ability to produce glutathione, which is considered the body's "Master Antioxidant". Antioxidant activity allows the body to get rid of the accumulated toxins and reduce inflammation. However, the administration of antipyretics, handcuffs the body from eliminating toxins which can lead to health complications like asthma, allergies, bronchitis, irritable bowel syndrome, chronic diseases, brain disorders, and even autism. Paracetamol is the leading cause of liver failure in the United States[28]. It has also been demonstrated that with an increase in paracetamol doses there is a corresponding increase in the cases of asthma and autism.

Paracetamol: Most Dangerous Compound in Medical Use Causes Acute Liver Failure

Study title: Acetaminophen/paracetamol: A history of errors, failures, and false decisions; *European Journal of Pain*[29], *November 2014*

From the abstract: Acetaminophen/paracetamol is the most widely used drug of the world. At the same time, it is probably one of <u>the most dangerous compounds in medical use</u>, causing hundreds of deaths in all industrialized countries due to acute liver failure (ALF). The history of the discovery of paracetamol starts with an error (active against worms), continues with a false assumption (paracetamol is safer than phenacetin), describes the first side-effect 'epidemy' (phenacetin nephropathy, drug-induced interstitial nephritis) and ends with the discovery of second-generation problems due to the unavoidable production of a highly toxic metabolite of paracetamol N-acetyl-p-benzoquinone imine (NAPQI) that may cause not only ALF and <u>kidney damage but also impaired development of the fetus and the newborn child</u>. It appears timely to reassess the risk/benefit ratio of this compound.

Reducing Fever with Paracetamol Increases Deaths by 5X in Patients with Critical Illness

Study title: The effect of antipyretic therapy upon outcomes in critically ill patients: a randomized, prospective study[30]; *Surgical Infections, 2005*

Objective of the study: To evaluate the impact of antipyretic therapy strategies on the outcomes of critically ill patients. Patients admitted to the Trauma Intensive Care Unit over a nine-month period were eligible for inclusion, except those with traumatic brain injury. Patients were randomized on day three of the ICU stay into aggressive or permissive groups. The aggressive group received acetaminophen 650 mg every 6 h for temperature of >38.5°C and a cooling blanket was added for temperature of >39.5°C. The permissive group received no treatment for temperature of >38.5°C, but instead had treatment initiated at temperature of >40°C, at which time acetaminophen and cooling blankets were used until temperature was <40°C. Patient demographics, daily temperatures, systemic inflammatory response syndrome (SIRS) scores, multiple organ dysfunction syndrome (MODS) scores, and infections and complications were recorded.

Results of the study: Between Dec 2002 and Sept 2003, 572 patients were screened, of whom 82 met criteria for enrollment. Forty-four patients were randomized to the aggressive group and 38 patients were randomized to the permissive group for a total of 961 and 751 ICU days, respectively. There were 131 infections in the aggressive group and 85 infections in the permissive group. <u>There were seven deaths in the aggressive group and only one death in the permissive group.</u> Study was stopped after the first interim analysis due to the mortality difference, related to the issues of waiver of consent and the mandate for minimal risk.

Conclusions of the study: <u>Aggressively treating fever in critically ill patients may lead to a higher mortality rate.</u>

Comment: So, you can see a huge difference in mortality. There were seven deaths in the group that administered antipyretics intensively, whereas only one death was in the group which did not use intensive drug therapy. It shows more than 5X times death.

Antipyretics like Paracetamol Increase Risk of Death by 30%

Study title: The effect on mortality of antipyretics in the treatment of influenza infection: systematic review and meta-analysis[31]; *Journal of the Royal Society of Medicine, October 2010*

Description: A systematic search of Medline, Embase and the Cochrane Register of Controlled Trials was undertaken to identify randomized placebo-controlled trials of antipyretic use in influenza infection in animal models or humans that reported mortality.

Results from the study: Eight studies from three publications met the inclusion criteria. No human studies were identified. <u>The risk of mortality was increased by antipyretic use in influenza-infected animals with a fixed effects pooled odds ratio of 1.34</u>. An increased risk was observed with aspirin, paracetamol, and diclofenac.

Paracetamol may not Improve Symptoms, but Prolong Illness as compared to Placebo

Study title: Acetaminophen: More harm than good for chickenpox? *The Journal of Pediatrics[32], June 1989*

Description: Study objective was to determine whether acetaminophen affects the duration or severity of childhood varicella. Seventy-two children between 1 and 12 years of age entered the study. 31 received placebo and 37 received acetaminophen. One child was withdrawn because of high fever, and three children did not complete the study.

Interventions: Acetaminophen, 10 mg/kg/dose, was given at 8 am, 12 pm, 4 pm, and 8 pm for 4 days. Placebo was given to the control group. Itching, appetite, activity, and overall condition were measured for 6 days. The time to last vesicle formation, time to total scabbing, and time to total healing were measured until complete resolution of the exanthem.

Measurements and main results: The following results were better in the placebo group: time to total scrabbing 5.6 days vs 6.7 days in the acetaminophen group and itching on day 4 in the placebo group symptom score 2.9 vs 2.2.

Conclusions of the study: These results provide evidence that acetaminophen does not alleviate symptoms in children with varicella and may prolong illness.

More Doses of Paracetamol Worsens the Illness in Children

Study title: Risks of antipyretics in young children with fever due to infectious disease[33]; *Acta Paediatrica Japonica, August 1994*

From the abstract: The objective of this study was to determine whether paracetamol (acetaminophen) affects the outcome of children with fever due to bacterial infectious disease. A total of 208 outpatients aged 6 months to 15 years with pyrexia due to bacterial infection who had been examined at the Fujimoto Children's Hospital from March 1992 to May 1992. The number of antipyretic doses of paracetamol (10 mg/kg) a day received within 3 days of illness in the patients with acute fever (> or = 38°C) was investigated. In this study, the patients were divided into two groups: (i) the pneumonia group, which consisted of 101 patients who were subsequently diagnosed as having pneumonia during their illness and (ii) the control group, which consisted of 107 patients who were subsequently diagnosed as having illness with fever that did not progress to pneumonia. The mean number of daily doses was significantly higher for the pneumonia group than for the control group.

There was no significant difference between the pneumonia group and the control group in body temperature during acute fever. The data suggest that frequent administration of antipyretics to children with infectious disease may lead to a worsening of their illness.

Paracetamol leads to Liver Related Complications

Study title: Effect of standard dose paracetamol versus placebo as antipyretic therapy on liver injury in adult dengue infection: a multicentre randomised controlled trial[34]; *The Lancet Global Health, May 2019*

From the abstract: Related observational studies in dengue have suggested that excessive paracetamol intake is related to hepatic injury. We aimed to evaluate whether standard dose paracetamol as an antipyretic in dengue infection caused transaminase elevation, and to evaluate the efficacy of paracetamol.

Methods: In this randomised, double-blind, placebo-controlled trial, adult participants (aged ≥18 years) with dengue, as confirmed by either positive NS1 antigen, positive dengue IgM antigen with thrombocytopenia, or positive PCR test, were enrolled at three Royal Thai Army hospitals in Thailand. Key exclusion criteria were baseline AST or ALT concentrations of more than 3 times the upper limit of normal, cirrhosis, indication of paracetamol other than dengue infection, concurrent diagnosis of other causes of fever, or pregnancy. Patients were randomly assigned by a computer-generated block randomisation procedure, to receive either paracetamol (500 mg) or placebo (500 mg) every 4 h when body temperature exceeded 38°C during hospitalisation. Participants and investigators were masked to treatment assignment. The primary outcome was the proportion of participants with transaminase elevation, defined as serum aspartate transaminase (AST) and alanine transaminase (ALT) concentrations of more than 3 times the upper limit of normal on recovery day, in the intention-to-treat population. Prespecified interim analyses for safety and efficacy were performed with group sequential stopping boundaries.

Findings: Between Sept 1, 2016, and Dec 12, 2017, 125 participants were randomly assigned to receive either paracetamol (n=63) or placebo (n=62). 123 participants were included in the intention-to-treat population. The median daily dose of study medication was 1·5 g. <u>The study was terminated early owing to a higher rate of transaminase elevation in the paracetamol group than in the placebo group</u> (22% vs 10%). The change of AST and ALT concentrations in the paracetamol group was higher than in the placebo group for ALT). Three participants in the paracetamol group had severe dengue: two had upper gastric haemorrhage and one had acute kidney injury. No patients died or had liver failure.

Interpretation: Use of standard dose paracetamol in dengue infection increased the incidence of transaminase elevation, and also overall transaminase concentrations in the absence of a counterbalancing reduced fever or pain score.

Paracetamol: Unsafe for Neurodevelopment in Children

Study title: Paracetamol (acetaminophen) use in infants and children was never shown to be safe for neurodevelopment: a systematic review with citation tracking[35]; *European Journal of Pediatrics, May 2022*

From the Abstract: Although widely believed by pediatricians and parents to be safe for use in infants and children when used as directed, increasing evidence indicates that early life exposure to paracetamol (acetaminophen) <u>may cause long-term neurodevelopmental problems</u>. Recent studies in animal models demonstrate that cognitive development is exquisitely sensitive to paracetamol exposure during early development.

The Effect of Paracetamol on Fever Clearance and Prevention of Seizures is not Superior to Placebo

Study title: Paracetamol for treating fever in children[36]; *The Cochrane Database of Systematic Reviews, 2002*

Description: The objective of the study was to assess the effects of paracetamol for treating fever in children in relation to fever clearance time, febrile convulsions, and resolution of associated symptoms in comparison to placebo (no treatment) and physical cooling methods.

Results: There is insufficient evidence to show whether paracetamol influenced the risk of febrile convulsions. The proportion of children without fever by the second hour after treatment did not differ significantly between those given paracetamol and those sponged (physical cooling method). <u>Trial evidence that paracetamol has a superior antipyretic effect than placebo is inconclusive.</u>

Paracetamol Overdose leads to Adverse Effects and Death

Study title: Estimates of acetaminophen (Paracetamol)-associated overdoses in the United States[37]; *Pharmacoepidemiology and Drug Study, June 2006*

Results of the study: Analysis of national databases show that acetaminophen-associated overdoses account for <u>about 56,000 emergency room visits and 26,000 hospitalizations yearly</u>. Analysis of national mortality files shows 458 deaths occur each year from acetaminophen-associated overdoses; 100 of these are unintentional.

Paracetamol does not Reduce the Chances of Seizures

Some people have the fear that a high fever could cause seizures. Yes, in rare cases there can be seizures, which might look very scary, however, they are usually benign and do not cause brain damage. Its prevention is difficult and may not be achievable[7]. Antipyretics cannot prevent Febrile seizures. There is now abundant evidence indicating that antipyretics have no effect on preventing further Febrile Seizures·

Study title: Do antipyretics prevent febrile convulsions?[38]; *Archives of Diseases in Childhood, July 2003*

From the article: Controlled studies of antipyretic medications, given during the original acute illness following a febrile seizure or during subsequent febrile episodes have failed to show a preventive effect in children at risk of FS. A recent review of trials assessing the effects of paracetamol on the clearance time of fever and on FS identified 12 randomised or quasi-randomised controlled trials. <u>It concluded that the trials failed to show any convincing evidence that paracetamol is effective in reducing fever or preventing FS.</u>

Paracetamol: May lead to Asthma in Children

Study title: The association of acetaminophen and asthma prevalence and severity[39]; *Pediatrics, December 2011*

From the Abstract: The epidemiologic association between acetaminophen use and asthma prevalence and severity in children and adults is well established. A variety of observations suggest that acetaminophen use has contributed to the recent increase in asthma prevalence in children

Maternal use of Painkillers (like Paracetamol) during Pregnancy is associated with Teratogenic Defects in Testicular Function and Gastrointestinal Tract

Study title: Intrauterine exposure to mild analgesics is a risk factor for development of male reproductive disorders in human and rat[40]; *Human Reproduction, November 2010*

Conclusion of the study: There was an association between the timing and the duration of mild analgesic use during pregnancy and the risk of cryptorchidism. These findings were supported by anti-androgenic effects in rat models leading to impaired masculinization. Our results suggest that intrauterine <u>exposure to mild analgesics is a risk factor for development of male reproductive disorders.</u>

Study title: Interindividual variability in acetaminophen sulfation by human fetal liver: implications for pharmacogenetic investigations of drug-induced birth defects[41]; *Birth Defects Research, March 2008*

Conclusion of the study: The results of this study lead to the hypothesis that <u>the mother's exposure to acetaminophen early in pregnancy is a risk factor for the development of gastroschisis in the offspring.</u>

Regular Use of Paracetamol is also linked with Certain Blood Cancers

Study title: Long-term use of acetaminophen, aspirin, and other nonsteroidal anti-inflammatory drugs and risk of hematologic malignancies: results from the prospective Vitamins and Lifestyle (VITAL) study[42]; *Journal of Clinical Oncology, June 2011*

Conclusion of the study: High use of acetaminophen was associated with an almost <u>two-fold increased risk of incident hematologic malignancies.</u>

Cases of Asthma Increase with the Increase in Sales of Paracetamol

Study title: Paracetamol sales and atopic disease in children and adults: an ecological analysis[43]; *The European Respiratory Journal, November 2000*

From the Abstract: Paracetamol sales were high in English-speaking countries, and were positively associated with asthma symptoms, eczema, and allergic rhino conjunctivitis in 13-14-yr-olds, and with wheeze, diagnosed asthma, rhinitis, and bronchial responsiveness in adults. <u>The prevalence of wheeze increased by 0.52% in 13-14-yr-olds and by 0.26% in adults for each gram increase in per capita paracetamol sales.</u>

Paracetamol Users have more Risk of Asthma

Study title: Acetaminophen and the risk of asthma: the epidemiologic and pathophysiologic evidence[44]; *Chest, Feb 2005*

From the Abstract: The prevalence of asthma has increased worldwide. The reasons for this rise remain unclear. Various studies have reported an association between acetaminophen, a widely used analgesic, and diagnosed asthma. In a prospective cohort study, the rate of <u>newly diagnosed asthma was 63% higher among frequent acetaminophen users than nonusers in multivariate analyses.</u>

A growing body of evidence over the last 5-7 years suggests that the use of paracetamol blocks the body's ability to produce glutathione, which is considered the body's "Master Antioxidant". When vaccines are taken, it commonly results in fever (as an attempt to detoxify the poisonous filth in vaccines). For example, 50–60% of young children develop fever after receiving the MMR vaccine[6]. To control this fever, parents often administer paracetamol to control the temperature. Paracetamol suppresses the fever by manipulation of the immune response. It reduces the body's ability to produce glutathione. It leads to a decreased ability to eliminate toxins and heavy metals such as mercury and aluminum found in vaccines. This also happens to a greater degree in genetically susceptible children that further prevents their bodies from eliminating the toxins.

Article title: Evidence that Increased Acetaminophen use in Genetically Vulnerable Children Appears to be a Major Cause of the Epidemics of Autism, Attention Deficit with Hyperactivity, and Asthma[45]; *William Shaw, November 2015*

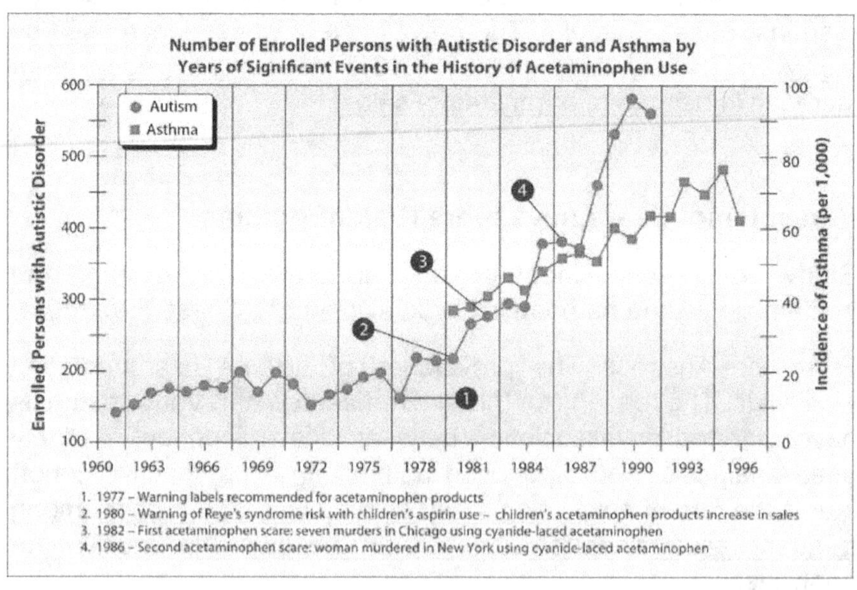

What can we understand from this graph? It shows that when the use of paracetamol increased, the cases of autism also increased (after 1977 and 1980). It also shows that when the use of paracetamol decreased, the cases of autism and asthma also decreased (after 1982 and 1986). The changes in the incidence of these very different diseases at exactly the time acetaminophen use dropped for a significant period of time is remarkable and may indicate the same factor as causing the asthma and autism[46].

It is not the acetaminophen that causes autism, rather its use in proximity to vaccination that appears to handcuff the body's ability to clear the metals and toxins. While it is true that many children that regress into autism do so without having been given this drug, it now appears that the drug may significantly increase that risk.

Paracetamol Interferes with Glutathione Production Reducing the Ability to Detoxify Metals and Toxins

Study title: The role of oxidative stress, inflammation, and acetaminophen exposure from birth to early childhood in the induction of autism[47]; *The Journal of International Medical Research, April 2017*

From the article: "The wide range of factors associated with the induction of autism is invariably linked with either inflammation or oxidative stress, and sometimes both. <u>The use of acetaminophen in babies and young children may be much more strongly associated with autism</u> than its use during pregnancy, perhaps because of well-known deficiencies in the metabolic breakdown of pharmaceuticals during early development. Thus, one explanation for the increased prevalence of autism is that increased exposure to acetaminophen, exacerbated by inflammation and oxidative stress, is neurotoxic in babies and small children." "This view mandates extreme urgency in probing the long-term effects of acetaminophen use in babies and the possibility that many cases of infantile autism may actually be induced by acetaminophen exposure shortly after birth." "Thus, it seems unwise to risk potentially permanent neurological injury for apparently ineffective pain relief."

Comment: This study emphasizes the fact that the bodies of babies and young children have difficulty in the metabolic breakdown of pharmaceuticals and toxins. One of the mechanisms that has repeatedly been shown is the fact that acetaminophen interferes with the body's production of glutathione, the most powerful detoxifying agent our bodies produce. This leads to a decreased ability to eliminate toxins and heavy metals such as mercury and aluminum found in vaccines. This is most likely one of the most important missing links in the autism discussion of causation. Couple a genetic susceptibility, with a drug that depletes glutathione given to relieve fever and pain caused by vaccine injection and it's a recipe for disaster.

Rat Pups produced Autistic Characteristics when Vaccinated with MMR and DPT and given Paracetamol

Study title: Effect of early natal supplementation of paracetamol on attenuation of exotoxin/endotoxin induced pyrexia and precipitation of autistic like features in albino rats[48]; *Inflammopharmacolog, Aug 2018*

The article strongly associated the connection with the development of autistic characteristics in rats that were vaccinated with MMR and DPT vaccines and given acetaminophen (Paracetamol-PCM), as is often done in human infants and children to control the fever from the vaccines.

From the Abstract: "The present study was aimed to test the hypothesis that paracetamol (PCM) can precipitate autistic like features when used to counteract vaccine-induced fever using experimental rat pups. The pups were treated with measles mumps rubella (MMR) vaccine, diphtheria tetanus and pertussis (DPT) vaccines and lipopolysaccharide (LPS) with subsequent PCM treatment. The pups were evaluated for postnatal growth (weight gain, eye opening) and behavior alterations (swimming performance, olfactory discrimination, negative geotaxis, nociception, and locomotor activity) by performing battery of neurobehavioral test. Significant correlation was observed between social behavioral domains (nociception, anxiety, and motor coordination) and pro-inflammatory load in the pups when treated with MMR/LPS along with PCM. A significant change in pro and anti-inflammatory (IL-4, IL-6, IL-10) markers were observed in rats treated with PCM, MMR, LPS, DPS alone or in combination with MMR, LPS and DPT."

(Note that significant changes were created in the IL cytokines that regulate inflammation with the vaccines alone and in combination with the PCM)

"Pups were also scrutinized for the markers of oxidative stress, inflammation and histopathologically. All the treatment groups showed significant alteration in the behavioral changes, oxidative markers, and inflammatory markers without following any specific treatment. This observation could be accorded to variable phenotypes (expressions) of autistic spectrum disorders (ASDs)."

Comments: <u>The markers of oxidative stress and inflammation were greater with the MMR + PCM, than the MMR alone. They were also greater with DPT + PCM, than with DPT alone.</u> This correlates with other similar studies and hypotheses that paracetamol interferes with the body's natural antioxidant and anti-inflammatory protective mechanisms. All the current vaccines are extremely toxic. And taking paracetamol after vaccination is extremely risky. It is especially harmful to those persons that have genetic defects in their ability to handle toxins already. Those are the ones at greatest risk of manifesting an autism spectrum disorder or a neurodevelopmental disability.

Study shows Autism and Paracetamol Connection

Study title: Acetaminophen (paracetamol) use, measles-mumps-rubella vaccination, and autistic disorder: the results of a parent survey[50]; *Autism, May 2008*

From the study: "The present study was performed to determine whether acetaminophen (paracetamol) use after the measles-mumps-rubella vaccination could be associated with autistic disorder. This case-control study used the results of an online parental survey conducted from 16 July 2005 to 30 January 2006, consisting of 83 children with autistic disorder and 80 control children. <u>Acetaminophen use after measles-mumps-rubella vaccination was significantly associated with autistic disorder when considering children 5 years of age or less</u>.

Comments: This preliminary study found that paracetamol use after MMR vaccine was associated with autistic disorder. Compared to controls, children ages 1-5 years with autism were eight times more likely to have gotten sick after the MMR vaccine and were six times more likely to have taken acetaminophen. Children with autism who regressed in development were four times more likely to have taken acetaminophen after the vaccine. Illnesses concurrent with the MMR vaccine were nine times more likely in autistic children when all cases were considered, and seventeen times more likely after limiting cases to children who regressed. This is important because acetaminophen (i.e., Tylenol or other brands), is often used to control fever after vaccination. Parents need to be aware of this serious risk and doctors need to stop recommending it. The results of this parent survey found a significant (600-800%) association with acetaminophen use after vaccination and autism.

What can we Conclude?

In the light of findings of the scientific studies, we can conclude that we do not need to fear a fever but allow it to run its course to support our life in various ways. Fever itself is not an illness. However, when a person gets a fever, there is an associated discomfort with it. However, as we discussed before, using antipyretics like paracetamol might reduce your body temperature and pain for some time, but it will also increase your chances of getting chronic diseases as well as damage your liver, kidneys, and immune system which will harm your long-term health. So, you might ask, "if we do not take any chemical-based drugs, then what is the natural and safe way to manage fever effectively?" Let us find out.

DISCLAIMER

The text, graphics, images, and other material contained in this book are for informational purposes only. No material in this book is intended to be a substitute for professional medical advice, diagnosis, or treatment. Always seek the advice of your physician or other qualified health care provider with any questions you may have regarding a medical condition or treatment and before undertaking a new health care regimen, and never disregard professional medical advice or delay in seeking it because of something you have read in this book.

Before we discuss the exact protocol that was recommended to the patients registered with Network of Influenza Care Experts (N.I.C.E) for management of Influenza like Illness, I would like you to read an analogy of a portable mobile charger. This analogy will help you understand the principle behind our recommended protocol of healing.

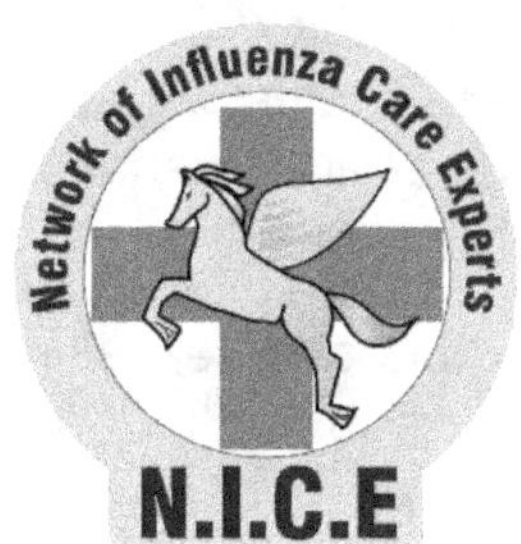

Think of your body as a portable mobile charger. If you try to charge three phones at a time, none of them will charge efficiently. But if you charge only one phone at a time, it'll charge quickly. Why? Because the charger has a limited source of power to distribute. It will charge more efficiently when it is catering to only one phone at a time. Similarly, every morning when you wake up, you get a limited source of energy. Every activity you perform - talking, walking, thinking, etc. consumes a little of this energy. By the evening, you feel tired because all of this energy has been consumed. When you sleep, you recharge yourself. When you eat something, your body's energy gets diverted into digesting it, leaving little for other tasks. That's why you feel sleepy after eating a heavy grain meal.

The fact of the matter is that your body can either spend the energy to digest or heal. If your body is digesting food all the time, it cannot heal properly. When you stop eating solids, you restrict the energy from going into digestion and divert it into healing. In the healing state, it cleans your liver, your kidneys, your colon, purifies your blood, helps you lose weight, flushes out the toxins and even reconstructs old scar tissue. So, during the happy diseases - symptoms of fever, cough, cold, etc., we must try to stop the consumption of solid food and try to fulfill our needs through fresh coconut water, vegetable soups, and freshly made juices of vegetables and fruits. By the fourth or fifth day, when you start feeling better, you can take fruits and raw vegetables in your diet and gradually resume with a healthy diet and lifestyle[51].

It is not as difficult as it might sound. When you fall sick, your taste buds change. You do not feel like eating food. You may remind yourself that Nature has taken away your hunger to allow your body a period of rest and healing. Even animals don't eat food when they're sick. They're more instinctive than us. When your dog falls sick, no matter how much food you give him, he won't eat till he's fine again. We have to adopt a similar practice in the case of Happy Diseases.

In this chapter, we will discuss the protocol that was followed by more than 60,000 patients in 2020-21 who were experiencing symptoms of fever, cough, breathing difficulty, diarrhea, headache, loss of smell and taste, etc. At that point of time, these symptoms were given the name of an imaginary new disease called 'Covid-19' caused by a fictitious 'SARS-CoV-2' virus[52]. It was a pre-planned conspiracy to inject the entire population with mRNA experimental vaccine from 2021 onwards.

The RT-PCR test is not a diagnostic tool, therefore, being 'positive' or 'negative' is irrelevant[53]. It does not matter that you have tested 'positive' or 'negative' for MERS, HIV, H1N1, Zika, Ebola, SARS-CoV-2, Monkeypox, Influenza A or B, C or D, etc. what matters is your symptoms, how you feel, what is the discomfort, and how to effectively manage it so that there are no future health complications, and you get normal and healthy in the safest and fastest manner.

The Covid-19 Plandemic was the biggest medical fraud of the decade. All the recommended measures to stop sickness were abject failure. Masks, sanitizers, social distancing, lockdowns, etc. were not only ineffective in reducing sickness but immensely disastrous to the natural health and immunity of the general population[54]. I have explained this in detail in the book "Do Face Masks Really Work?". These irrational measures also caused burden on the economy and proved to be an environmental hazard. The Covid-19 vaccine propaganda was pushed by the nexus of government, pharmaceuticals, politicians, crisis actors, media houses and medical establishments. Most of the people fell for the lies and took the experimental vaccine. This led to massive adverse reactions to millions of people across the world[55].

I have been informing the public about the vaccination agenda of the pharmaceutical companies from the beginning of 2020. It was similar to the previous medical frauds like HIV AIDS. The restrictions that were imposed on the population in the name of health were catastrophic. It made people submit to the unscientific, irrational, and harmful advice of the so called "medical experts". The masks do not stop or prevent a "viral" disease[56]. However, they are excellent for psychological operation on the minds of the population. Constant wearing of masks by every person served as a constant reminder that a fatal disease was spread all around in air. It kept the fear instilled in every mind and heart. The sanitizers were harmful for natural immunity and skin health. The lockdowns were to keep the society disintegrated and shut down small businesses (and make them financially dependent on the government). Social distancing caused feeling of loneliness in people that led to high amounts of stress and affected natural immunity[57].

The Covid-19 vaccine is completely ineffective in stopping or preventing cough, cold, diarrhea, etc. (so called symptoms of Covid-19). However, it has the potential to cause numerous side effects which took 9 pages for Pfizer to list together in a document titled Cumulative Analysis of Post-authorization Adverse Event Reports.[58] (See page no. 30 to 38)

I am a member of Network of Influenza Care Experts (N.I.C.E) founded and trained by Dr. Biswaroop Roy Chowdhury. This network was built to support the people in natural healing from symptoms of Influenza like Illness as people were excessively scared. The 72-hour liquid diet protocol was given to all the patients who registered in our portal and within 3 to 7 days, all the patients recovered well and got back to normal work life by following the protocol. This was a voluntary service which was provided free of cost and the results were phenomenal. It was successful at curing all the patients with no money, no medicines, and no mortality. Thousands of people could recover easily from the so called 'deadliest' virus in the history of mankind with this protocol. I was fortunate to serve and care for more than 250 patients as an expert in the network of influenza care. I was honored with the title of 'Corona Warrior' from Indo-Vietnam Medical Board for my service.

So, let us now come to the solution. As soon as the first signs and symptoms of flu are experienced, like feeling feverish, headache, body ache, cold, cough, etc., immediately stop eating solid foods and start following the 72-hour liquid diet protocol. The 72-hour liquid diet protocol is extremely effective and is based on collective evidence from multiple research papers[59]. Citrus fruits are rich in Vitamin-C and boost immunity. Coconut water maintains the mineral balance and gives hydration to the body. Cucumber and tomatoes are rich in vitamins, fibre, and contain plenty of water.

72-HOUR LIQUID DIET PROTOCOL

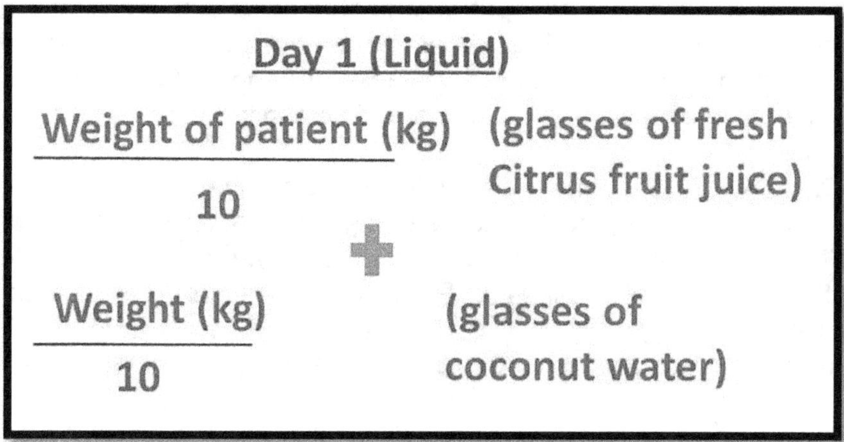

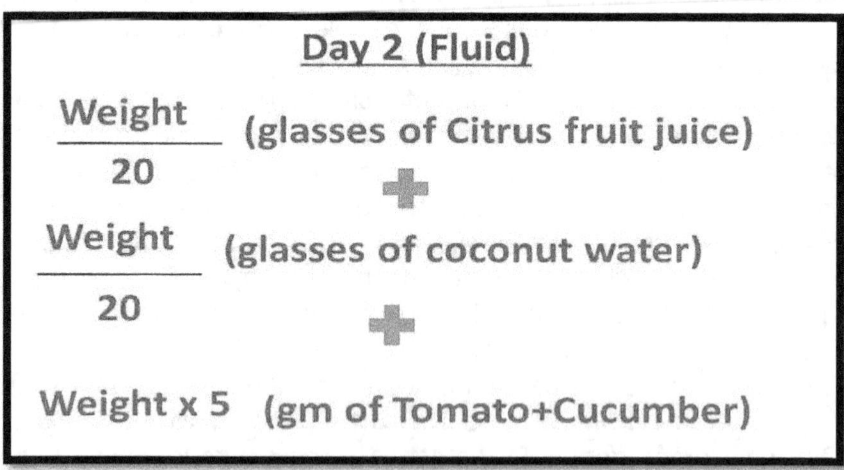

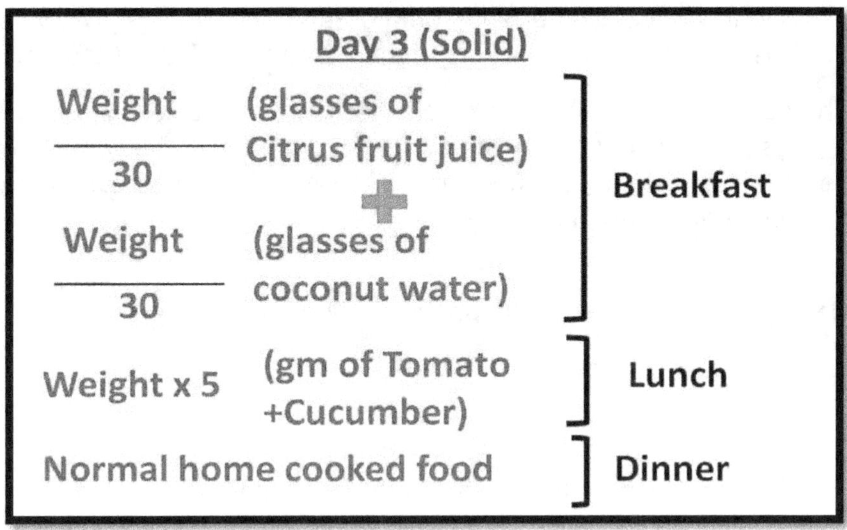

Let us say that a patient gets a fever on some day. His weight is 60 kgs. To begin the process of natural healing through our protocol, he must stop eating solid foods and start following the 72-hour liquid diet protocol in the following manner:

Day 1: Follow the routine as per instructions below:

1. Glasses of citrus fruit juice = Weight (kgs) ÷ 10
    Glasses of citrus fruit juice = 60 ÷ 10 = 6 glasses

2. Glasses of coconut water = Weight (kgs) ÷ 10
    Glasses of coconut water = 60 ÷ 10 = 6 glasses

The person is required to drink 6 glasses of fresh coconut water and 6 glasses of freshly made citrus fruit juice on day 1.

Day 2: Follow the routine as per instructions below:

1. Glasses of citrus fruit juice = Weight (kgs) ÷ 20
    Glasses of citrus fruit juice = 60 ÷ 20 = 3 glasses

2. Glasses of coconut water = Weight (kgs) ÷ 20
    Glasses of coconut water = 60 ÷ 20 = 3 glasses

3. Quantity of Cucumber and Tomato Salad = Weight (kgs) x 5
    Quantity of Cucumber and Tomato Salad = 60 X 5 = 300 grams

The person is required to drink 3 glasses of fresh coconut water and 3 glasses of freshly made citrus fruit juice on day 2. Besides that, he may consume about 300 grams of a raw vegetable salad made from cucumbers and tomatoes.

Day 3: Follow the routine as per instructions below:

Breakfast:

1. Quantity of citrus fruit juice = Weight (kgs) ÷ 30
    Quantity of citrus fruit juice = 60 ÷ 30 = 2 glasses

2. Quantity of coconut water = Weight (kgs) ÷ 30
    Quantity of coconut water = 60 ÷ 30 = 2 glasses

Lunch:

1. Quantity of Cucumber and Tomato Salad = Weight (kgs) x 5
    Quantity of Cucumber and Tomato Salad = 60 X 5 = 300 grams

Dinner:

1. Home cooked vegetarian meal without oil and minimum salt

The 72-hour liquid diet protocol resulted in complete recovery of most of the patients registered with Network of Influenza Care Experts within 3 days. However, if complete recovery is not achieved in 3 days, then the 72-hour liquid diet protocol can be repeated one more time. Once, the body temperature comes in normal range, then the diet recommended for day 3 can be repeated for 2-3 more days and then a healthy and balanced diet can be resumed.

The most important thing while managing Flu / ILI / Covid-19 is managing the symptoms like breathing, fever, cough, vomiting, nausea, and extreme weakness. In such a situation, the person might panic; we need to remind them that they need to keep some patience; that is why they are called patients. Only two things are mainly important: the temperature and the oxygen saturation level (SpO2). As long as the temperature is ≤102°F, it is not harmful and there is no need to worry. Remember, there is no scientific evidence that a fever below 104°F can cause serious damage to the body[7]. Also, if the oxygen saturation level is ≥ 90% during sickness, then it is not at all harmful and there is no need to worry.

1. Fever Management

There is no need to worry as long as the fever is equal or less than 102°F (≤ 102°F). If the temperature crosses 102°F, along with the 72-hour liquid diet protocol, you must also start the process of wet packs (cold compress) and fan with cold air for 15 minutes.

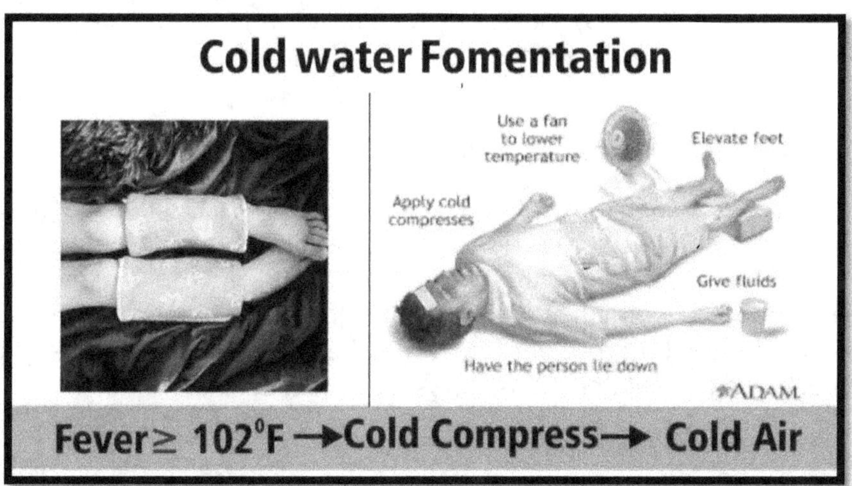

To do wet packs (cold compress): Take 3 to 5 cotton cloths. Soak them in cold water and squeeze them out. Now wrap the wet pack around your stomach, neck, head and/or both calf muscles.

If the patient starts shivering, stop the process (it is an indication that the body does not want to have the temperature reduced at that point of time). After a gap of half an hour, repeat the wet packs (cold compress) and fan cold air for 15 minutes. If he starts shivering or if the temperature comes down to 101.5°F, stop the process.

In some cases, the temperature rises to 103°F - 104°F, do not panic in such a situation. Panic or stress will never solve the problem. You might feel that I should take an antipyretic drug, but ask this question, will reduction in the temperature with antipyretic drug also enhance my quality of life, increase my chances of survival, and benefit my long-term health? Remember, antipyretics may reduce the temperature for some time, but as per scientific evidence it does not reduce the chances of seizures or death. There is inconclusive evidence that paracetamol or any antipyretic drugs can help a person to survive better, live a longer life, or to avoid the seizure in comparison to not taking the antipyretic drugs.

Even if temperature gets very high, don't panic because our body has its own homeostasis and will not let the temperature be dangerously high. It knows at what temperature the toxins can be eliminated, or any harmful pathogen can be killed (if that is assumed to be cause of illness). However, keep providing cold compress and cold air and continue to follow the 72-hour liquid diet protocol.

2. Breathing Management:

You could check the SpO2 with the help of an Oximeter. If the reading is ≤ 88%, there is a chance of breathlessness. If the patient was in a hospital, a situation of SpO2 ≤ 88% would mean an emergency according to the hospital staff and the patient would be recommended to be put on a mechanical ventilator. What is mechanical ventilator? What does it do? Is it safe?

The mechanical ventilator is something big, looks very scientific, something very promising, something very glamorous in a way that it is very expensive and not everyone can afford. People assume that it is a marvellous product of modern medical science. People believe that a hospital with big equipment has a greater ability to save a person's life, but it is a belief only, not the reality.

A mechanical ventilator means a pipe goes from a machine to your nose and mouth to the lungs and stomach. It is a bedside machine with tubes that connect to your airways. It is supposed to "help" you take breaths if you can't do it on your own. A ventilator mechanically pumps purified oxygen into your body. The air flows through a tube that goes in your mouth and down your windpipe. The breathing tube is extremely uncomfortable. While it is hooked up, you can not eat, drink, or talk.

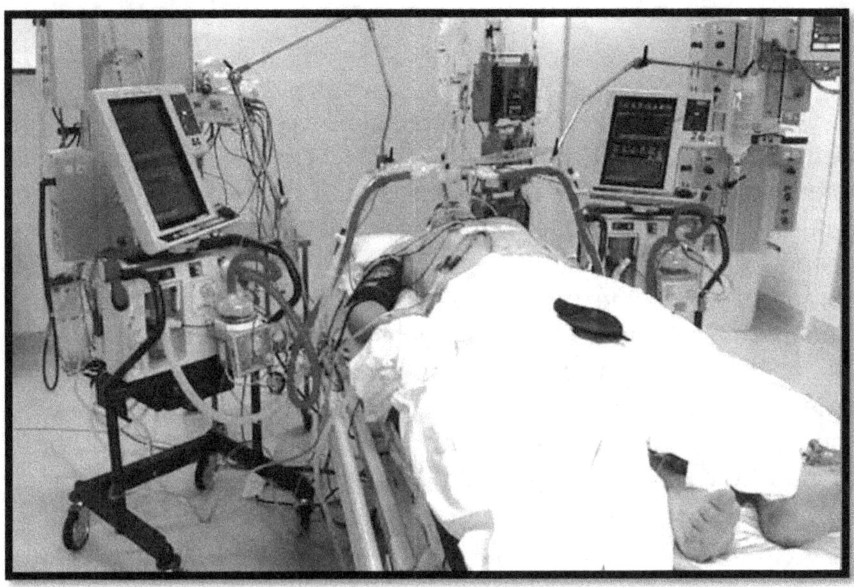

When too may pipes go into the body, they give rise to many complications. It is observed that majority of the patients who are put on the ventilator never come back from the ventilator. Only rare patient survives, it might not be because of the ventilator but he survives in spite of being put on the ventilator. So, the patient may be called lucky or extremely unlucky. Lucky because he survived a dangerous machine. Unlucky because staying on the ventilator is very painful. Those who come out are in a miserable state and their lifespan is greatly reduced. According to K. B. Tumane MD, a retired senior medical officer, a specialist in the lungs department, he never saw a patient come back alive from the mechanical ventilator in his entire career. What makes the mechanical ventilator so dangerous?

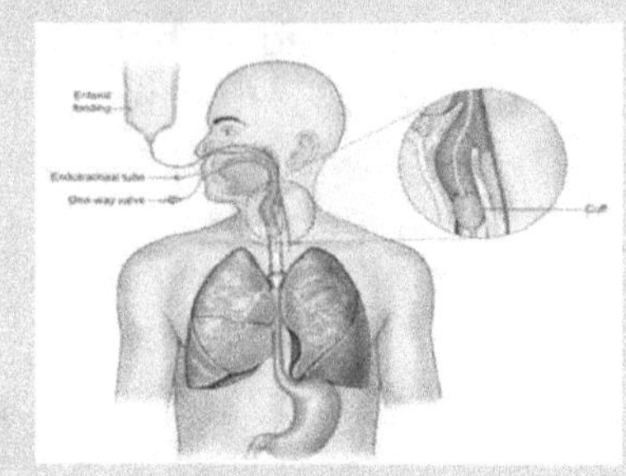

1. When the patient is on a mechanical ventilator, he might get Ventilator Associated Lung Injury (VALI). Concentrated oxygen is forced on the lungs at a particular speed. Since our body is not naturally designed to take the stream of purified oxygen at any speed, it damages the lungs gradually, which were already compromised in the first place. For evidence, you can read the Cochrane Systematic Review[60] in which two groups of people were taken: one group was given higher concentration of oxygen and the other group was given lower concentration of oxygen. Those who were given oxygen with higher concentration suffered more harm; those who received oxygen with lower concentration suffered less harm. So lower concentration of oxygen is better.

Higher v/s Lower Oxygen

Higher versus lower fraction of inspired oxygen or targets of arterial oxygenation for adults admitted to the intensive care unit

Cochrane Systematic Review – 27 November 2019

2. Putting the patient on a mechanical ventilator may cause oxygen toxicity. Our body is not designed to continuously intake pure oxygen but breathe air, a mixture of gases, through the nose. However, the ventilator forces purified oxygen in the lungs of the patient which may result in oxygen toxicity.

3. The speed and the concentration of oxygen forced in the lungs may cause neuro-damage. The brain and the lungs, which ordinarily work in coordination, might start losing the harmonious connection with each other after the person is put on the ventilator. As a result, the person has diminished memory and has difficulty to perform regular life skills, only if he manages to come out alive from the machine.

4. In extreme cases, the person might suffer from Ventilator Associated Pneumonia (VAP). When a number of pipes go into your body, the bacteria and virus travel through the pipe and occupy a place in the inner part of the lungs. This is called Ventilator Associated Pneumonia and can lead to death.

The Solution: Prone Ventilation

Conclusion of a Randomised Control Trial study published in New England Journal of Medicine: "In patients with severe Acute Respiratory Distress Syndrome (ARDS), early application of prolonged prone-positioning sessions (of 16 hours) significantly decreased 28-day and 90-day mortality[61]."

So, when the patient feels breathless or his SpO2 level drops below 90%, ask the patient to lie down in prone position for an hour and again check the SpO2 and you will find it would have increased by 1-2% and the patient will also start feeling better. How does it work?

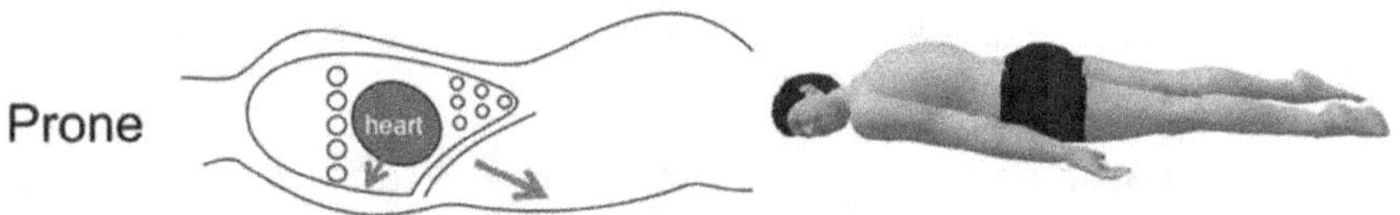

The prone position alters the mechanics and physiology of gas exchange to result consistently in improved oxygenation. The improvement of oxygenation during prone ventilation is multifactorial. Prone positioning improves gas exchange by ameliorating the ventral-dorsal transpulmonary pressure difference, reducing dorsal lung compression, and improving lung perfusion[62,63].

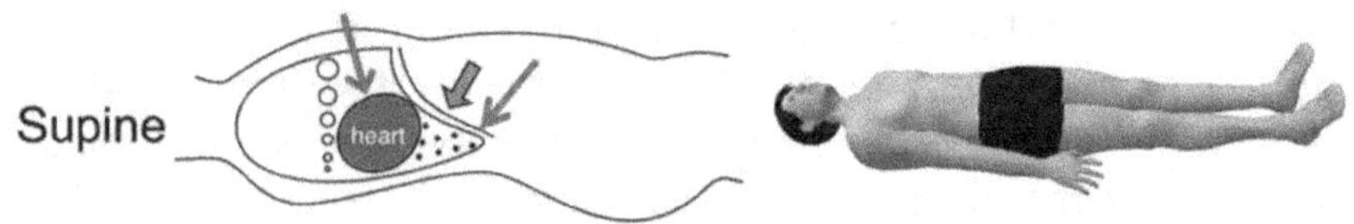

We normally lie down (with face up). The small dots represent the sacs/alveoli. In this position, the pressure of heart and the pressure of abdomen lie on the corner of the lungs and as a result, the balloons squeeze in size thereby about 20% capacity of the lungs is reduced. A healthy human has no effect with the 20% reduction in the lungs capacity but when one is sick (since 20% is compromised), it has a visible effect.

If we can take away the pressure of the heart and the abdomen, then we can utilize that 20%. For this, we need to change the posture, it is called prone positioning or prone ventilation. As you can see, the small balloons become bigger in size, and this increases the capacity of the lungs by about 20%. The person, who was believed to on the verge of death earlier, now has some chances of survival with natural and safe method.

Prone ventilation has been in practice since 1970s. In the last one decade or so, when the mechanical ventilator became popular, prone ventilation and other such things were sidelined to promote the sale of mechanical ventilator. Prone ventilation has no side effects as compared to the mechanical ventilator[64]. On one hand is mechanical ventilator which is expensive, painful, and dangerous and on the other hand is prone ventilation, which is safe, effective, free of cost, and can be done at home.

In order to make the patient more comfortable in the Prone ventilation position, a pillow can be placed as shown in the picture, since some people have big bellies. The big belly may compress the lungs as a result you may not get the advantage of 20%. How to adjust the pillow can be decided by the comfort level of the patient. Motivate the patient to be in this position for 12-16 hours to get the most advantage. This is how one can manage the breathing at home.

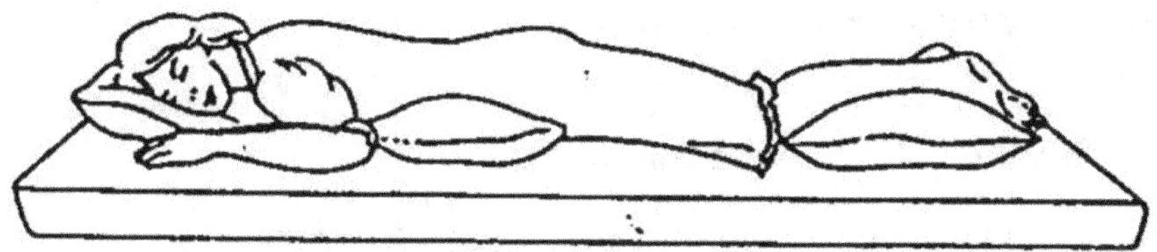

To conclude, when you put a person on Prone ventilation, the abdominal as well as the heart pressure are less, there is increased alveolar capacity and thus improved breathing. All this is expected to start in about half an hour. But here the recommendation is that the patient should be in Prone ventilation posture for at least 12 to 16 hours in a day because the moment he gets up, the breathing problem might start again. So, he may take a break of 10-15 minutes every hour. During the break, he can move his body and be in any posture.

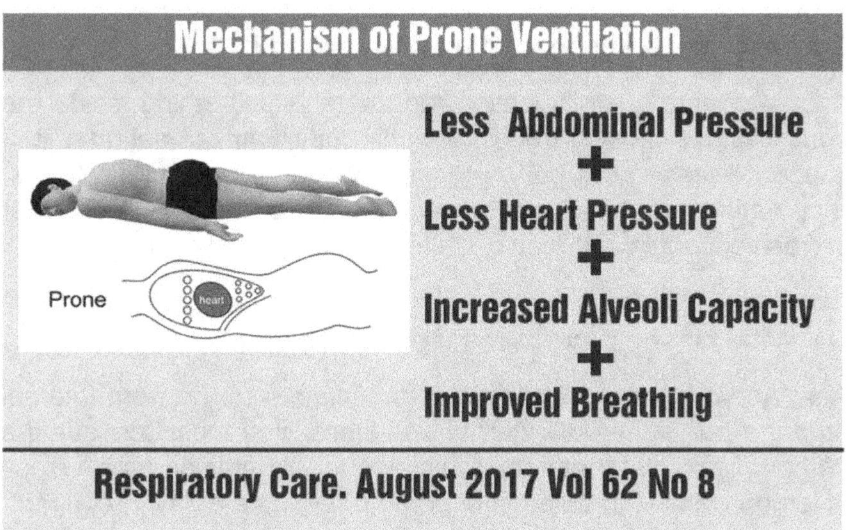

Frequently Asked Questions:

Q1. What can be done to manage cough?

Ans: You may reduce the quantity of citrus fruit juices by 50% and consume a small piece (5 gm) of raw turmeric three times a day. If you aren't able to do the turmeric therapy, you may drink a cup of decoction of ginger and black pepper twice a day.

Q2. What can be done to manage diarrhea?

Ans: If loose motions occur more than 5-6 times in a day, then you should stop consuming everything, and only take fresh water or fresh coconut water as and when required till loose motions subside or completely stop. Wet packs (cold compress) with a cotton cloth around the stomach can also be done for 15 mins 3 times in a day.

Q3. What can be done to manage vomiting?

Ans: Vomiting is an indication that there is something inside the body which is causing trouble and the body wants to get rid of it. It is not a disease itself but a process trying to throw out the toxins. Stop eating and drinking everything for 4 to 6 hours. Simple water or fresh coconut water can be taken as and when required.

Q4. What can be done to manage weakness?

Ans: As your energy is diverted to eliminate toxins from internal organs, you might feel external weakness. You must continue the 72-hour liquid diet protocol. You may eat 2-3 dates or drink a glass of lemon water with a spoon of pure honey twice a day if required.

Q5. What can be done to manage body pain?

Ans: To relieve your body of some pain, you may place both of your legs in a bucket of hot water with temperature above 40°C (or the temperature which is bearable yet hot). This can be done twice or thrice a day. You must continue the 72-hour liquid diet protocol.

Q6. Which juices can be taken as a citrus fruit juice?

Ans: Oranges, pineapples, kiwis, etc. are some common examples of citrus fruits. You may prepare fresh juices from them. It is advised that you consume the juices within 15 minutes of preparation.

Q7. Can we take a hot vegetable soup on day 1 or day 2?

Ans: A clear vegetable soup is permissible once a day in 72-hour liquid diet protocol. You may boil all seasonal vegetables in water; strain it; add salt, pepper, and lemon; consume it slowly while hot.

Q8. Can we consume herbal hot decoctions?

Ans: You may consume freshly made hot herbal decoctions twice a day. These are recommended in cases of fever, cough, cold and headache. You can boil 2-3 black pepper, ¼ tsp cinnamon, 2-3 cloves, and 1-2 gm ginger in water. Strain the liquid and drink it while hot. Drink it slowly, sip by sip, while inhaling the vapours.

Q9. Shall I continue my medicines during the 3-day fast?

Ans: For anyone who is on medication, we always recommend that you consult your medical doctor about how to adjust your medicine dosage during the 72-hour liquid diet protocol. There might be a need to adjust your medications, so it is best to connect with your trusted medical doctor for advice.

Q10. How much water should I drink?

Ans: There is no fixed amount of water that we must consume throughout the day as it varies from person to person based on multiple factors. Always remember - you must listen to your body and drink water when you're thirsty. Sometimes, your requirement of water may go down as the fresh juices are very hydrating and fulfil the requirement of liquids in our body and as we are not consuming cooked food, so there is no intake of items like salt, spice, oil, or refined sugar which tend to dehydrate us. Preferably, you may take warm water when needed and consume it slowly.

Q11. Can I do 3-day water fast instead of 72-hour liquid diet protocol?

Ans: Water fasting has been suggested by many healers and it has positive results in most cases. However, water fasting is much more advanced than juice fasting. If you have never fasted before, we suggest that you start with 72-hour liquid diet protocol, as it is a more gradual approach. If you are used to fasting and have completed several fasts before, you may do a 3-day water fast. Please ensure to take sufficient rest throughout the day if you are water fasting. Do not do any strenuous mental or physical work.

Q12. Can someone who has a chronic disease like type-2 diabetes or hypertension follow the 72-hour liquid diet protocol?

Ans: I cannot give a personal medical advice for what a patient with chronic disease do as every case can be different on many parameters, however, the 72-hour liquid diet was used by N.I.C.E on thousands of patients who were on diabetic medication or hypertension medications. They all recovered well, the only thing you must ensure is to monitor your blood sugar and blood pressure levels continuously and adjust the medication dose with the help of your medical doctor as there may be fluctuations in blood sugar or blood pressure while on 72-hour liquid diet protocol.

Q13. What things are recommended to support the 72-hour liquid diet protocol?

Ans: Make sure that the juices are freshly made, and no salt should be added to them. Drink them slowly - each glass should take at least 5 minutes to drink. Proper physical and mental rest is of immense value. Sleep in a well-ventilated room. Avoid watching television, using phone, and working on computer. Switch off the Wi-Fi in the house. Spending few minutes in mild sunshine is beneficial. Doing few minutes of simple pranayama like alternative nostril breathing on an empty stomach can be useful. Simple exercises or stretching can be performed for few minutes. Do not engage in heavy lifting or exertion.

You must maintain a positive attitude and offer your prayers to the supreme healing power, Almighty God. Sexual activity must be stopped for the period of healing as it leads to overstimulation of your senses, which prevent you from getting adequate sensory rest.

Q14. Who will take the responsibility if someone in our family does not take anti-pyrectics during fever and dies?

Ans: Do you think that the thousands of the people who die every year with influenza like illness, are not given antipyretics like paracetamol? Does the hospital take the responsibility of the patient's death? Does the doctor take the responsibility of the patient's death? People die even while they are given anti-pyretic drugs. Shockingly, according to the available evidence there is greater chances of death by consumption of antipyretics as compared to placebo (or no treatment). The truth is that every physical body on earth will die and finish one day, and no human is immortal. Decision about the treatment is patient's responsibility.

You have to take the decision based on your rational thinking by studying the evidence. Always ask this question to your doctor, "Is there evidence that by taking the drug or therapy being offered by you, I will be able to enhance my quality of life, or increase my span of life in comparison to taking no treatment at all?" You will realise that most of the drugs and therapies offered by the hospitals do not have evidence to give a favourable answer to this question.

There is data of 60,000+ patients who recovered from ILI without medications by following the 72-hour liquid diet protocol under the supervision of Network of Influenza Care Experts in 2020-21. Ultimately, every person is responsible for his own decisions and actions. In the upcoming section you will be shocked to see the statistics that how mistakes by hospital staff and adverse drug reactions are a leading cause of death in the world. In spite of the available evidence, in spite of being proven that multiple therapies, drugs and treatments provided by the hospitals are extremely toxic and fatal, they are still continuing. Who will take the responsibility to raise questions on those toxic drug therapies? People must wake up and start asking questions to those who push poisonous therapies like chemotherapy, radiation therapy, vaccinations, etc.

Should vaccines really get credit for the decline of infectious diseases?

Most practising doctors and nurses undoubtedly believe that vaccines have helped wipe out some of the deadliest infectious diseases. Many members of the medical profession would put vaccination high on any list of great medical discoveries. Those who promote vaccines often claim that vaccination programmes have reduced illness and prevented millions of deaths. These are all barefaced lies. This simply is not true; it is a myth.

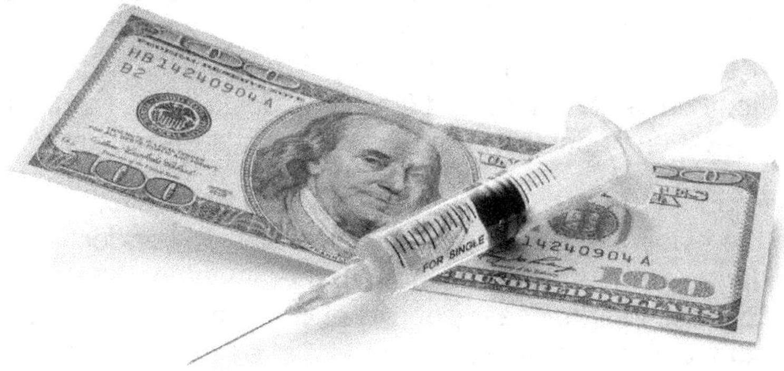

The introduction of vaccination programmes came along either just at the same time or later when the death rates from the major infectious diseases had already fallen. The evidence shows that the diseases which are supposed to have been wiped out by vaccines were disappearing long before vaccines were introduced. It shows that vaccination programmes have not done the things they are credited with but have done most of the things they are blamed for.

The reason that most of these diseases were decreasing already was the significant improvements that were made in personal hygiene, improved sanitation habits, refrigeration, sewage elimination, better nutrition, and cleaner water supplies during the last hundred years.

Anyone who doubts this has to only look at graphs showing mortality rates and life expectation rates alongside graphs showing when vaccines were introduced. The graphs show clearly that the improvements took place before the vaccines were introduced. Study the evidence related to whooping cough, tetanus, diphtheria, smallpox, and other diseases and it becomes clear that the incidence of these diseases, and number of deaths caused by them, were in decline long before the relevant vaccines were introduced[65].

The graph on the next page depicts that the mortality for several common illnesses had already declined significantly long before the vaccines were created. The downward trend of the curves is completely unaffected by vaccine introduction[66].

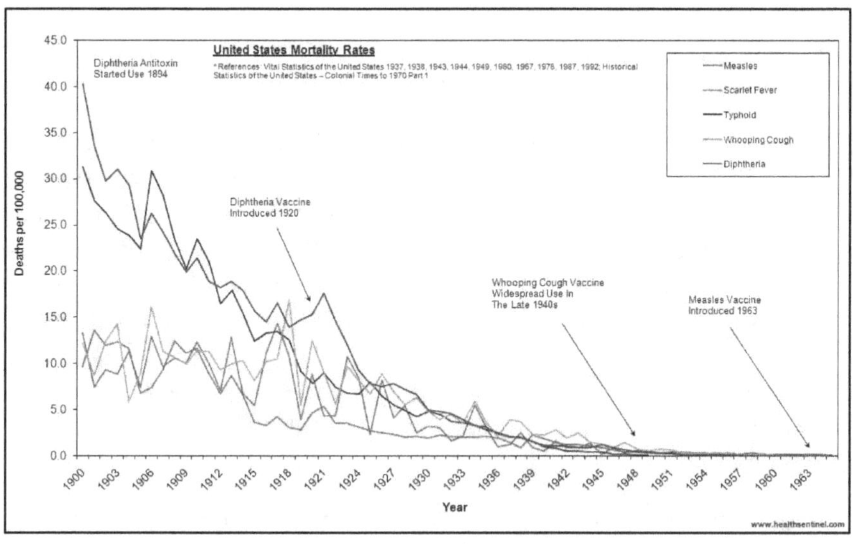

In recent history in underdeveloped and third-world nations, we have seen rates of infectious disease similar to what they used to be in western countries 100 years ago, prior to all these improvements. And yet, many of these impoverished nations are seeing dramatic improvements in hygiene, sanitation, better nutrition, and clean water. Also, the rates of infectious disease complications and deaths are also dropping significantly.

So, how do they fool the masses? A vaccine is introduced, and the trajectory of the disease goes down. The most important question that no one ever asks is, what was the trajectory of the disease before the vaccine was introduced? If the trajectory of disease was declining before the vaccine was introduced, it is probable that the vaccine got the credit for something it did not do.

The principle behind vaccination is a convincing one. The theory is that when an individual is given a vaccine - which consists of a weakened or dead version of the disease against which protection is required - his or her body will be tricked into developing antibodies to the disease in the same way that a body develops antibodies when it is exposed to the disease itself. But things aren't quite so simple. How long do the antibodies last? Do they always work? What about those individuals who do not produce antibodies at all? What about the adverse effects from the ingredients of the vaccine? What about the deaths and permanent disabilities caused to some of the vaccine recipients?

After spending countless hours on vaccine research: studying thousands of research papers, reading hundreds of books, watching dozens of censored documentaries, interviewing dozens of medical doctors, and meeting with children who suffered vaccine injuries, I concluded that vaccines are ineffective, unsafe and may cause serious health complications like ADHD, learning disabilities, behavioral challenges, neurological deficits, autism spectrum disorders, allergies, eczema, asthma, autoimmune conditions, type 1 diabetes, rheumatoid arthritis, obesity, cancer, reproductive and thyroid issues and even death.

I would not be taking any of the vaccines for myself. This is a personal view, and it is not a view shared by most doctors, nurses, and journalists. Those who are reading this book must make their own judgements and decisions based on all the available evidence. The bottom line is that I do not advise anyone to not take a vaccine. I do not advise anyone to take a vaccine. I do not advise anyone to vaccinate or not vaccinate their child. My role, as a writer, is to provide information which is not being provided by the Government or the medical profession.

LATEST: A study published in November 2020 reveals that the children who never took any vaccine are much healthier than the children who took all the vaccines!

For many years, vaccine educated people and organizations have been asking the CDC, WHO, pharmaceutical companies, and other relevant governmental agencies to do comparison studies looking at the health status, frequency of doctor's visits, and hospitalizations of children that have been vaccinated and those that have not been vaccinated. They have all refused to conduct such studies till now. Thankfully, recently some studies have been done by outstanding independent. Here we look at some of those brilliant studies without conflict of interest and industry bias.

Study title: Relative Incidence of Office Visits and Cumulative Rates of Billed Diagnoses Along the Axis of Vaccination[67]; *International Journal of Environmental Research and Public Health, November 2020*

Description: This study categorizes the illnesses that vaccinated and unvaccinated children went for doctor's office visits during their first nine and a half years of life. It is a peer-reviewed study that shows clearly that unvaccinated children are healthier than vaccinated children.

From the Abstract: Increased office visits related to many diagnoses were robust to days-of-care-matched analyses, family history, gender block, age block, and false discovery risk. Many outcomes had high RIOV odds ratios after matching for days-of-care (e.g., anemia (6.334), asthma (3.496), allergic rhinitis (6.479), and sinusitis (3.529), all significant under the Z-test)."

"Remarkably, zero of the 561 unvaccinated patients in the study had attention deficit hyperactivity disorder (ADHD) compared to 0.063% of the (partially and fully) vaccinated. The implications of these results for the net public health effects of whole-population vaccination and with respect for informed consent on human health are compelling. Our results give agency to calls for research conducted by individuals who are independent of any funding sources related to the vaccine industry."

Conclusions of the study: "We could detect no widespread negative health effects in the vaccinated other than the rare but significant vaccine-targeted diagnosis. <u>We can conclude that the unvaccinated children in this practice are not, overall, less healthy than the vaccinated and that indeed the vaccinated children appear to be significantly less healthy than the unvaccinated.</u>"

The following table shows the Relative Index of Office Visits for the fully vaccinated (N1 = 2763) vs. never vaccinated (N2 = 561).

Condition	Vaxxed	Unvaxxed	RIOV	95% CI	Z	p
Fever	759	17	9.065	8.801	12.476	<0.0001
"Well Child" Visits	32,826	4987	1.336	1.149	6.540	<0.0001
Ear Pain	269	16	3.414	3.232	5.310	<0.0001
Otitis media	3105	216	2.919	2.518	23.441	<0.0001
Conjunctivitis	1018	87	2.376	1.935	9.783	<0.0001
Eye Disorders (Other)	277	31	1.814	1.586	3.350	0.0008
Asthma	336	13	5.248	5.065	6.693	<0.0001
Allergic Rhinitis	405	12	6.853	6.662	8.158	<0.0001
Sinusitis	107	5	4.345	4.240	3.566	0.00036
Breathing Issues	621	44	2.866	2.561	7.898	<0.0001
Anemia	979	36	5.522	5.181	13.603	<0.0001
Eczema	512	23	4.520	4.281	8.479	<0.0001
Urticaria	174	17	2.078	1.908	3.027	0.00244
Dermatitis	742	105	1.435	0.992	4.034	<0.0001
Behavioral Issues	343	17	4.097	3.900	6.087	<0.0001
Gastroenteritis	688	30	4.656	4.374	6.543	<0.0001
Weight/Eating Disorders	1115	90	2.515	2.056	10.264	<0.0001
Seizure	43	8	1.091	0.985	0.229	0.8181

RIOVs were calculated using the number of patients as the sample size in each group (Vaxxed and Unvaxxed) with the exception of well-child visits and otitis media visits, both of which were greater in number than the number of patients.

What can we understand from the above table? The above table portrays that that the vaccinated group of children has relatively about 6 times more episodes of allergic rhinitis, about 5 times more episodes of asthma, about 5 times more episodes of anemia, about 4 times more episodes of sinusitis, about 4 times more episodes of eczema and about 9 times more episodes of fever besides increased risk of all other diseases like ear and eye disorders, stomach disorders, behaviour disorders, etc. It would not be wrong to say that vaccinated children are sicker in all parameters as compared to children who never took any vaccines.

You may read in detail about the hidden truth of vaccinations in my #1 Best Seller book in epidemiology and infectious diseases titled 'The Vaccine Crime Report'.

From the initial chapters of this book, it is clear that symptoms like cough, cold, fever, diarrhea, etc. which are common to every infectious disease are actually mechanisms of self-cleansing. These are not necessarily caused by a virus like H1N1, COVID-19, Zika, SARS, MERS, Influenza, Monkeypox, etc. These are categorized as influenza-like illnesses in the medical industry. So, what are we trying to stop with the flu shots and why?

We need answer to three main questions. First of all, is stopping symptoms like cough, cold, fever, etc. beneficial for our health in the long term? Secondly, does the vaccine really stop these symptoms? Thirdly, what about the side effects of flu shots? Let's look at the relevant scientific studies to understand these:

Flu Shot did not Reduce Flu Cases in Children but Caused a Higher Rate of Other Respiratory Illness within 14 days

Study title: Assessment of temporally-related acute respiratory illness following influenza vaccination[68]; *Vaccine, April 2018*

Description: The study found that children who are vaccinated for influenza develop a higher rate of non-influenza acute respiratory illness in the 14 days after the vaccination than those that are not vaccinated.

Results from the study: "The hazard of influenza in individuals during the 14-day post-vaccination period was similar to unvaccinated individuals during the same period."

Conclusion of the study: "Among children there was an increase in the hazard of ARI (Acute Respiratory Illness) caused by non-influenza respiratory pathogens post-influenza vaccination compared to unvaccinated children during the same period."

Influenza Vaccines may Increase the Risk of Influenza

Study title: Association between the 2008—09 seasonal influenza vaccine and pandemic HINI illness during Spring— summer 2009: four observational studies from Canada[69]; *PLoS Medicine, April 2010*

Description: Four studies showed that recipients of a seasonal influenza vaccine had a significantly increased risk of subsequently developing severe pandemic influenza (H1N1) compared to people who did not receive the seasonal vaccine.

The Influenza Vaccine May Increase the Risk of Other Respiratory Infections by 4x

Study title: Increased Risk of Non-influenza Respiratory Virus Infections Associated with Receipt of Inactivated Influenza Vaccine[70]; *Clinical Infectious Diseases, June 2012*

Description: The study challenges the thinking that immunization against the flu reduces flu symptoms such as upper respiratory infections. The reality is that vaccination against the flu appears to increase the rates of other non-influenza upper respiratory infections by greater than 400%!

From the study: "We randomized 115 children to trivalent inactivated influenza vaccine (TIV) or placebo. Over the following 9 months, IV recipients had an increased risk of virologically confirmed non-influenza infections." "TIV recipients may lack temporary non-specific immunity that protected against other respiratory viruses."

Influenza Vaccine completely Ineffective in Children

Study title: Influenza vaccine effectiveness among children 6 to 59 months of age during 2 influenza seasons: a case-cohort study[71]; *Archives of Pediatrics and Adolescent Medicine, October 2008*

Conclusion of the study: "In 2 seasons with suboptimal antigenic match between vaccines and circulating strains, we could not demonstrate VE (Vaccine effectiveness) in preventing influenza-related inpatient/ED or outpatient visits in children younger than 5 years."

Hospitalisation Risk Increases by 3x in Children after Influenza Vaccine

Report title: Flu Vaccination May Triple Risk for Flu-Related Hospitalization in Children with Asthma[72]; *American Thoracic Society, May 2009*

Description: The report looked at children over a 10-year period who did and did not receive the flu vaccine. It was determined that children that got the flu vaccine were 3 times more likely to be hospitalized than those that were not vaccinated.

From the report: "In order to determine whether the vaccine was effective in reducing the number of hospitalizations that all children, and especially the ones with asthma, faced over eight consecutive flu seasons, the researchers conducted a cohort study of 263 children who were evaluated at the Mayo Clinic in Minnesota from six months to 18 years of age, each of whom had had laboratory-confirmed influenza between 1996 to 2006. The investigators determined who had and had not received the flu vaccine, their asthma status and who did and did not require hospitalization. Records were reviewed for each subject with influenza-related illness for flu vaccination preceding the illness and hospitalization during that illness.

"<u>They found that children who had received the flu vaccine had three times the risk of hospitalization, as compared to children who had not received the vaccine.</u> In asthmatic children, there was a significantly higher risk of hospitalization in subjects who received the Trivalent Influenza Vaccine, as compared to those who did not."

A 2018 Cochrane Review of 52 Studies on the Effectiveness of the Influenza Vaccine in over 80,000 Healthy Adults shows that being Vaccinated Maybe only 1% better than not being Vaccinated

Study title: Vaccines for preventing influenza in healthy adults[73]; *The Cochrane Database of Systematic Reviews, February 2018.*

From the study: "Healthy adults who receive inactivated parenteral influenza vaccine rather than no vaccine probably experience less influenza, from just over 2% to just under 1% (moderate-certainty evidence)." "71 healthy adults need to be vaccinated to prevent one of them experiencing influenza."

Fifteen included trials were industry funded (29%). This is interesting. What I mean by that is, if nearly a third of the studies they looked at were funded by the drug industry (and you can bet they put their best numbers forward), and that didn't even skew the results in their favor, most likely the non-drug industry studies found even less or no benefit at all.

So, one must ask himself, is it worth playing Russian Roulette with all the toxic ingredients from the flu vaccine to have negligible benefit at all? Why not just optimize the vitamin and mineral levels, eat healthy, get quality sleep, practice good hygiene and we could lower the risk much more than risking the injection of flu shot. People often hold the misconception that the current medical system is the best and the medical doctors and hospitals are working their best to keep the population healthy. However, the truth is completely opposite, and I am trying to bring it out.

To know the dark reality of the other popular vaccines like Hep-B, Polio, MMR, DTaP, HPV, etc., you may read my #1 Best Seller book in epidemiology and infectious diseases titled 'The Vaccine Crime Report'. In the next section you would get a glimpse of the statistics that will showcase the immense failure of the current medical system around the world.

An Interesting Tale of a Medical Class (Allopathy)

Good morning, students! Today I welcome you all to the first day of medical college and you are going to learn about the medicine, and we are going to start with hypertension or high blood pressure. There are several medicines, but we are going to talk about a medicine called diuretics which is considered very safe. The discomfort is very less, and it is almost safe and effective.

There are a few side effects of **Diuretics** such as erectile dysfunction, impotency, abnormal rhythms, palpitations, nausea, vomiting, headache, dizziness, joint pain, lethargy, tiredness, weakness but there is no need to worry. If a patient complains of erectile dysfunction, **Viagra** can be given but even after taking Viagra there are a few side effects like weakness, headache, dizziness, running nose, indigestion, etc. If a patient complains of headache after taking Viagra, he can be given **Paracetamol**. Even Paracetamol may lead to liver failure, constipation, or allergy, for which some other medicine can be provided.

The doctors have a solution for every problem in the form of medicine. For instance, for indigestion, **Zantac** can be recommended. Even after Zantac, a patient may complain of insomnia, diarrhea, nausea, or constipation, but again some medicine can be recommended. In the same way, for a person suffering from abnormal rhythm, **Pronestyl** can be given which may result in diarrhea or loss of appetite. If he complains of loss of appetite, he can be given **Imodium**. However, some side effects of Imodium are constipation, dizziness, abdominal pain, vomiting and nausea.

Diuretics	Viagra	Paracetamol	Zantac	Pronestyl
Impotency	Indigestion	Constipation	Constipation	Bitter taste
Joints pain	Runny nose	Allergy	Insomnia	Weakness
Weakness	Weakness	Liver failure	Weakness	Headache
Headache	Headache	Jaundice	Headache	Nausea
Nausea	Backache	Nausea	Nausea	Dizziness
Palpitations	Redness	Diarrhea	Diarrhea	Diarrhea
Dizziness	Dizziness	Stomach pain	Dizziness	Appetite loss

So, in this way, the list of medicines keeps increasing and at the end of the day, the patient himself forgets the problem for which he had initially consulted the doctor. He just remembers the medicines to be taken in the morning, afternoon, and night. He starts taking medicines as food and feels that he is protected because of these medicines. This is enough for you to understand that the patient is now going to drown in a whirlpool of problems[4]. He can only be saved by his due diligence.

Another Problem with the Germ Theory

Let us try to understand the above through the analogy of a banana peel. You will understand why the medical industry has failed to address the real cause of disease, thus failing to reach the true cures.

One morning, you wanted to eat a banana. So, you took off the peels and ate the edible part of it. Now, it's the time to throw the peels. If you do not throw the banana peel out into the garbage bin, but instead put it on your kitchen table, in a short period of time, banana flies will start to feast on it. However, if you throw the banana peel into an effectively managed dustbin, the flies will disappear quickly.

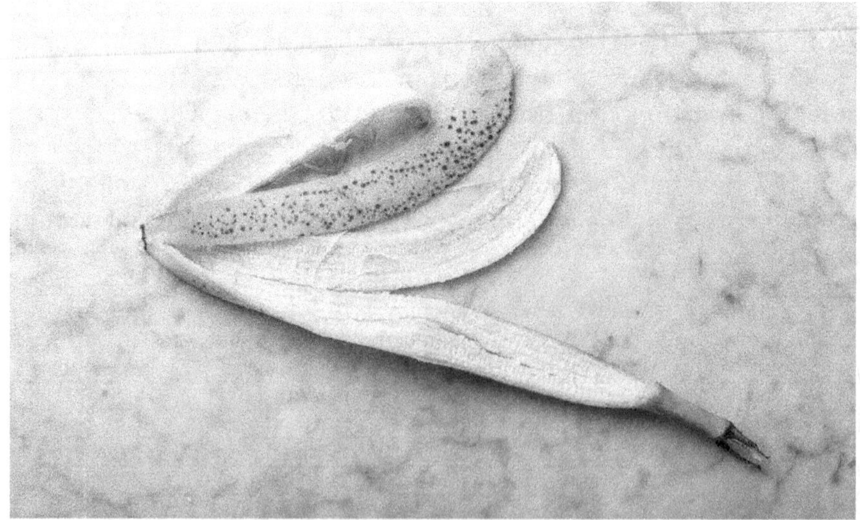

This means that the decomposing banana peel was the cause of the infestation of banana flies. If you remove the banana peel, they will not have anything to eat and will fly away to try to find another source of food or they will simply die. Of course, you could kill the flies, but without removing the banana peel you would only see new ones coming in. Same goes for micro-organisms, they are usually not the main cause of disease, but can give you a hard time if they get a chance to proliferate beyond your body's ability to cope with them. What conclusions can we draw from this example?

Well, keep your inner environment clean and in balance and the micro-organisms living in the body will work for you, not against you. They will not give you a hard time, because you do not interfere with nature. Many of them are actually necessary for you and will help you to maintain good health. If we learn how to live according to the laws of nature, we do not have to fear the micro-organisms. The best prevention of disease is living a healthy lifestyle according to the laws of nature.

However, the real prevention of disease (living a healthy lifestyle) is unfortunately not taught at medical schools. The dogma of the germ theory of disease is pushed to all the medical students. It can sometimes be dangerous because they almost always see germs as the causative agents and treat the disease with antibiotics which does not help but often only makes things worse.

Evidence of Harms caused by Hospitals and Drugs

The current medical system is far from being safe. Medical researchers have continued to highlight the lower safety of the medical profession. An important example is the number of people that die due to medical error in hospitals every year. In 1999, the prestigious Institute of Medicine, published a report titled 'To Err is Human'. Dr Lucian Leape MD, a Harvard pediatrician who is referred to as 'the Father of Patient Safety' was on the committee that wrote the report. The report was published in the Journal of the American Medical Association (JAMA) and shocked the medical world. It stated that 98,000 people die annually due to medical mistakes in hospitals[74].

Another report titled 'Is US Health Really the Best in the World?' was published in Journal of the American Medical Association (JAMA) in July 2000 by Barbara Starfield MD. It states that the health care system contributes to poor health of Americans through its adverse effects. For example, every year United States estimates about 12000 deaths from unnecessary surgery, 7000 deaths from medication errors in hospitals, 20000 deaths from other errors in hospitals, 80000 deaths from nosocomial infections in hospitals and about 106000 deaths from adverse effects of medications. <u>These total to 225000 deaths per year from iatrogenic causes which becomes the third leading cause of death in the United States, after deaths from heart disease and cancer</u>[75]. Can you imagine that the medical system itself to be the third leading cause of death in the United States?

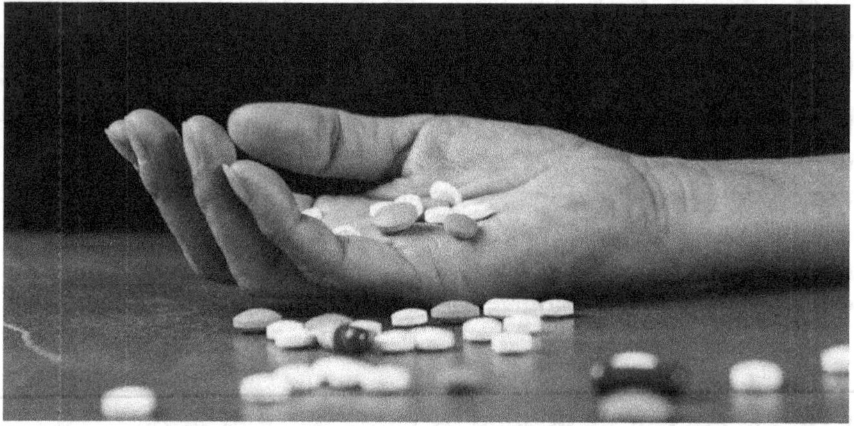

After a few years, a group of researchers thoroughly reviewed the statistical evidence and their findings on medical errors were shocking. Gary Null PhD authored a paper titled 'Death by Medicine' that presents powerful data that today's medical system often causes more harm than good. This fully referenced report demonstrates <u>the number of people having in-hospital, adverse reactions to prescribed drugs to be 2.2 million per year</u>. The number of unnecessary antibiotics prescribed annually for viral infections is 20 million per year. The number of unnecessary medical and surgical procedures performed annually is 7.5 million per year.

The number of people exposed to unnecessary hospitalization annually is 8.9 million per year. <u>The most stunning statistic, however, is that the total number of deaths caused by conventional medicine is an astounding 783,936 per year</u>[76]. It might be somewhat correct to say that the medical system, itself, can be considered as the leading cause of death and injury in the United States. (It exceeds the number of deaths attributable to heart disease 699,697 and cancer 553,251 as per the statistics.)

Unfortunately, the news has continued to get worse since then. An article published in the Journal of Public Safety September 2013 titled, 'A New Evidence-based Estimate of Patient Harms Associated with Hospital Care', found that a minimum of 210,000 preventable deaths per year occur in the U.S. and that the number may exceed 400,000 because of the limitations of the search tools they used. Incredibly, they also determined that serious harm to patients in hospitals may be 10-20 times greater than that horrific lethal number of 400,000! <u>That means between 4 million and 8 million people are seriously harmed in hospitals annually in the U.S!</u>[77]

According to a 2016 article published in the Journal of Community Hospital Internal Medicine Perspectives, titled the alarming reality of medication error: a patient case and review of Pennsylvania and National data, there is a dangerous and costly number of medication errors annually in the U.S.

"Errors occurred at multiple care levels, including prescribing, initial pharmacy dispensation, hospitalization, and subsequent outpatient follow-up. This exemplifies the Swiss Cheese Model of how errors can occur within a system. <u>Adverse drug events (ADEs) account for more than 3.5 million physician office visits and 1 million emergency department visits each year</u>[78]. It is believed that preventable medication errors impact more than 7 million patients and cost almost $21 billion annually across all care settings. About 30% of hospitalized patients have at least one discrepancy on discharge medication reconciliation. Medication errors and ADEs are an underreported burden that adversely affects patients, providers, and the economy.

What do the above Statistics tell us?

This shows that the medical industry has absolutely failed in the prevention and treatment of illness, sickness, and disease. More and more people are going to visit doctors than ever before. More and more people are getting diagnosed regularly through blood tests, X-rays, ultrasounds, etc. than ever before. More people are taking pills and drugs than ever before. There are more surgeries performed than ever before. But still, more people suffer from diseases like diabetes type-2, heart disease, hypertension, thyroid imbalance, polycystic ovarian syndrome, obesity, multiple sclerosis, asthma, bronchitis, sinusitis, chronic kidney disease, ulcers, piles, acid reflux, constipation, cancer, etc. The only winners in the medical system are the healthcare and drug companies. The drug companies' profits are skyrocketing. The medical industry has no genuine interest in the prevention and curing of any illness but their own profits.

In my personal experience with hundreds of people with the above conditions, I have seen that majority of these diseases that have been termed as incurable, are reversible and also curable within a few months by eliminating the cause of the disease by following a regimen of natural diet and lifestyle that has the potential to activate self-healing mechanism of the body. Anyone who is ready to eradicate the root cause of their disease will successfully recover if they un-do what caused the disease and start doing what heals it. You can read more about such natural cures in my book 'Advanced Nutrition Therapy: Goodbye Drugs and Diseases' or visit my website 'https://gosatvik.ca/mystory' to watch the testimonial videos of the patients healed through natural nutrition therapy[79].

An ideal scenario would be waking up in the morning full of energy, vitality, content, and feeling blessed. You enjoy your day with energy, a bounce in your step, a smile on your face. You don't feel stressed, anxious, or depressed; you don't feel tired, you have no headaches or pain in your body; you are not overweight, and your skin is glowing. You have a good appetite and eat what you want, and you are never that hungry. You don't deprive yourself of the foods you enjoy. You go to sleep at night, and you sleep soundly and peacefully and get a wonderful whole night's rest. Your skin, your hair, and your nails look healthy and radiant. You have strength and tone in your muscles. Your body is fluid, graceful, and flexible. You are firm, strong, vibrant, and feel great! These are the signs of a healthy person.

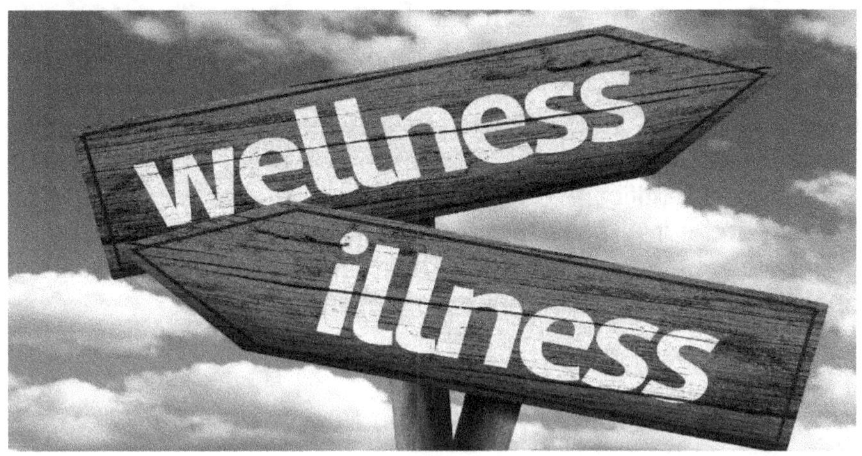

A healthy person rarely needs to take a drug. A healthy person never has to have surgeries. Being sick is not "normal," it is abnormal. Most people think they are healthy, but they really have no idea just how much better they could feel. A healthy person has no cancer, diabetes, or heart disease. A healthy person lives without illness, sickness, or disease. Most people have no idea how good their body is designed to feel. We have been brainwashed into believing that it is natural for a human being to have aches and pains, and have major medical problems like cancer, diabetes, and heart disease. We are also brainwashed into believing that it's "natural" to take drugs. We are programmed to believe that we "need" drugs in order to be healthy.

Is there a place for surgery and drugs? The answer is absolutely yes! Medical science has done a decent job at addressing symptoms. However, the treatment of a symptom has two flaws. First, the treatment itself usually causes more problems which will have to be treated later. Second, the cause of the symptom is usually never addressed. When you do not address the cause, you are allowing for problems later on.

With this said, if you are in an emergency situation such as that caused by a sudden accident of some sort, drugs and surgery can save your life. However, drugs and surgery have failed at preventing illness and they do not address the cause of illness. Nevertheless, they do work well (not always) in most emergency crisis situations. The bottom line is, if you fall off a ladder and puncture an organ, you want to be rushed to the closest emergency room and have a trained medical doctor use drugs and surgery to save your life. But if you want to stay healthy and never have disease, drugs and surgery are not the answer. So, if trillions of dollars in scientific research have failed in producing ways to prevent and cure illness and disease, and all-natural inexpensive prevention methods and cures do exist, why aren't we hearing about them? The answer may surprise you.

What if the Cure is Discovered and People are made Aware?

Imagine there is a scientist working in a lab somewhere[80]. He makes a breakthrough discovery: A small plant is found in the Amazon that, when made into tea and consumed, eliminates all cancer in the body within one week. Imagine this researcher proclaiming that he has given this tea to one thousand cancer patients and that every single one of them, within one week and without having undergone surgery, was found to have absolutely no cancer in their body. Eureka! A cure for cancer! A simple, inexpensive, all-natural cure with no side effects. Just a simple plant that you make into tea and drink. It has absolutely no side effects at all. It's pure, all-natural, and costs just a penny.

Imagine this scientist announcing his discovery to the world. Certainly, he would win a Nobel Prize. Certainly, the world medical community would be rejoicing. No more cancer! Every cancer patient could drink this tea and in one week be free of all their cancer. Every person who lives with the fear of getting cancer could now know that they could simply drink a few cups of this tea, which costs them only a few pennies, and they could avoid ever getting cancer. The world would be a better place.

Unfortunately, you'll never hear this story. Not because the story is not true, but because if this simple herbal tea which cures all cancer was allowed to be sold, there would be no need for the American Cancer Society. There would be no need for any of the drug companies that are manufacturing and selling cancer drugs. There would be no need for any additional cancer research funding. Cancer clinics around the world would close, hundreds of thousands of people would be put out of work, entire industries would shut down overnight and billions and billions and billions of dollars in profit would no longer be funneling into the kingpins who control the cancer industry.

So, when this person makes this discovery, what happens? In some cases, these people simply vanished. In other cases, these people were given hundreds of millions of dollars for their research. In still other cases the federal government raided these researchers' offices, confiscated the data, and jailed the researchers for practicing medicine without a license. Is this fantasy or is this the truth? Well, the health-care industry has a dirty little secret, and I am blowing the whistle on it. We all must take responsibility for our own health. We have to become our own doctor, own nutritionist, own healer, and own therapist.

My books are written to impart to you the required knowledge based on experience and evidence. It will assist you to remain free from the clutches of experimental drugs and therapies, to successfully reverse your chronic illnesses and confidently go through the process of happy diseases. My latest book "Do Face Masks Really Work" contains all the evidence that the current medical industry is a puppet of the tyrannical forces that wish to bring the Great Reset or the New World Order. It provides you a roadmap of their plan and suggests various measures that we can take to protect ourselves and our loved ones from the coming challenges.

72-HOUR LIQUID DIET PROTOCOL

Day 1 (Liquid)

$$\frac{\text{Weight of patient (kg)}}{10} \quad \text{(glasses of fresh Citrus fruit juice)}$$

$$+$$

$$\frac{\text{Weight (kg)}}{10} \quad \text{(glasses of coconut water)}$$

Day 2 (Fluid)

$$\frac{\text{Weight}}{20} \quad \text{(glasses of Citrus fruit juice)}$$

$$+$$

$$\frac{\text{Weight}}{20} \quad \text{(glasses of coconut water)}$$

$$+$$

$$\text{Weight} \times 5 \quad \text{(gm of Tomato} + \text{Cucumber)}$$

Day 3 (Solid)

$$\left.\begin{array}{l}\dfrac{\text{Weight}}{30} \quad \text{(glasses of Citrus fruit juice)} \\[4pt] + \\[4pt] \dfrac{\text{Weight}}{30} \quad \text{(glasses of coconut water)}\end{array}\right\} \text{Breakfast}$$

$$\left.\text{Weight} \times 5 \quad \text{(gm of Tomato} + \text{Cucumber)}\right\} \text{Lunch}$$

$$\left.\text{Normal home cooked food}\right\} \text{Dinner}$$

21 HEALING STORIES (2020-21)

(Our clients who followed 72-hour liquid diet protocol)

1. Kawaljeet Singh from Mumbai tested positive for Covid-19 on 12th October 2020. He was prescribed about 15 (experimental) tablets by the medical` doctor. He felt breathlessness. He was not 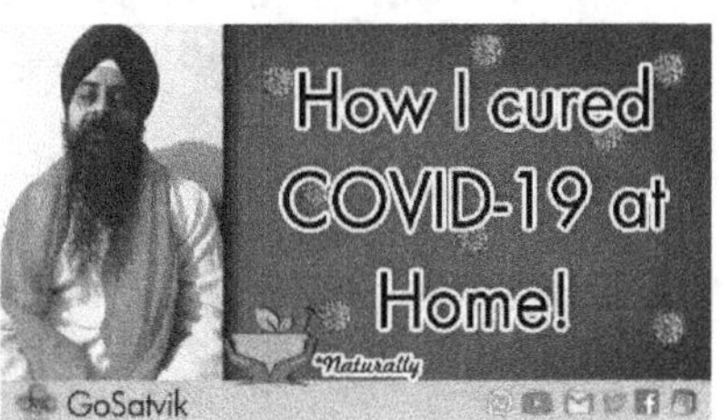

able to sleep with constant headaches and vertigo. He reported to Dr. Singh on the recommendation of his friend. He had fever of 103.5°F and symptoms of cough and cold. His family was in panic. Dr. Singh gave them strength and hope. He advised them to follow the 72-hour liquid diet protocol and do wet packs to manage temperature. He got fully normal on the 3rd day. He tested negative for Covid-19. He did not consume any drugs. He says my belief in natural cures has increased.

2. Monika from Maharashtra tested positive for Covid-19 and reported to Dr. Singh with symptoms of fever. Her daughter aged 8 months had a temperature reach up to 103°F. The family did not 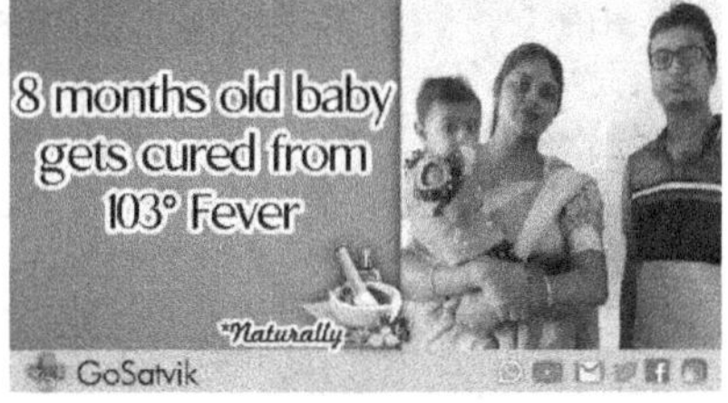

consume any drugs and followed the 72-hour liquid diet protocol. The 8 months old child was given her mother's milk and a limited quantity of coconut water and fresh orange juice. She was normal in 3 days and all symptoms were gone. They did not take paracetamol even when everyone was pressurizing them. They used wet packs to manage the temperature.

3. Manoj from Chandigarh reported to Dr. Singh about his father who had extreme breathlessness, and SpO2 level was 61%. The family was very scared, and they were aware that during Corona 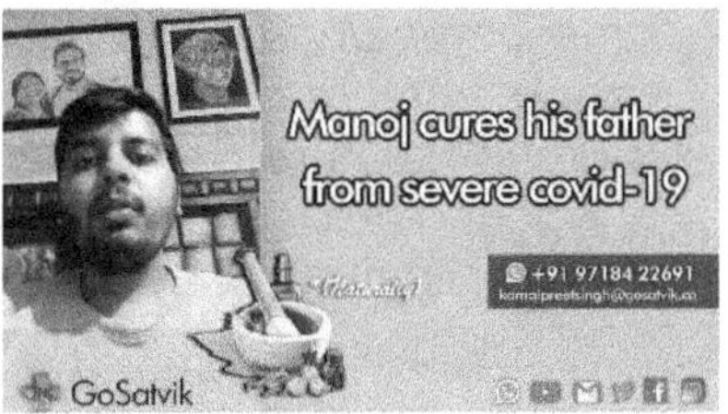

Plannedemic the hospital would give fatal experimental drugs like remdesivir, favipiravir, etc. to his father and charge huge money. They followed the 72-hour liquid diet protocol on the recommendation of Dr. Singh and did Prone Ventilation at home for 12+ hours regularly. He feels that his father is alive today because of the timely support received through Dr. Singh.

4. Ganesh Dilwale, age 36 yrs., had the symptoms of fever and weakness on 20th September 2020. He was tested positive for Covid-19. He kept consuming paracetamol for 1 week according to medical doctor's

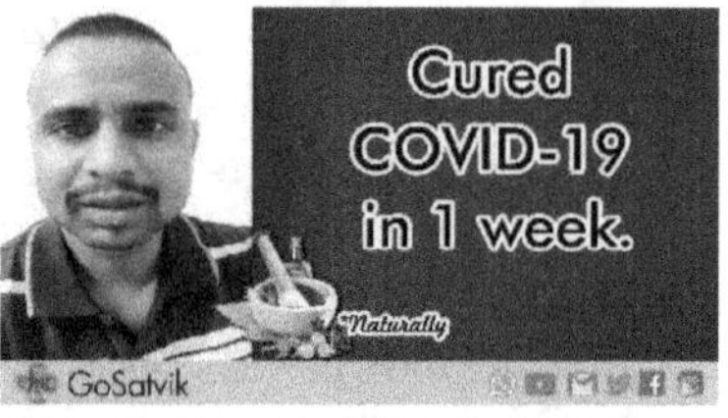

advice, but no relief was seen. He reported to Dr. Singh and his weakness and fever were gone within 24 hours of following the 72-hour liquid diet protocol. He did not consume any drugs. He says that he is now aware of the scam of Covid-19. He also tested negative for Covid-19 later.

5. Saurabh Mishra from New Delhi, age 27 yrs., tested positive for Covid-19 on 9th September 2020. He took paracetamol and azithromycin for 3 days, but no relief was seen. He stopped the drugs and reported to Dr. Singh

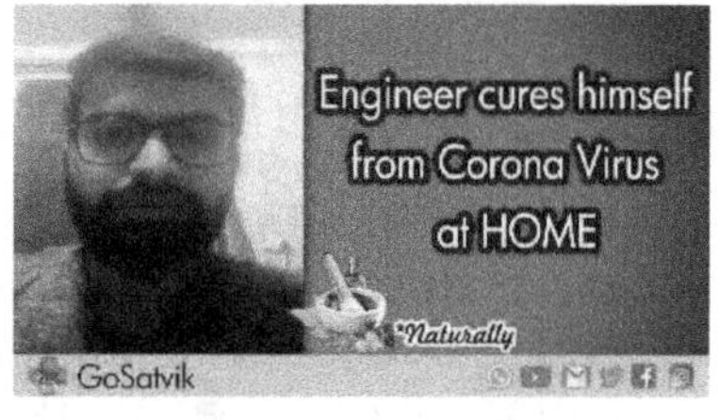

and followed the 72-hour liquid diet protocol. Within 3 days, he was cured and tested negative for Covid-19 the next week.

6. Sukhwinder Singh from New Delhi, age 27 yrs., tested positive for Covid-19 with symptoms of fever, cough, weakness, and loss of smell. He took paracetamol for some days along with cough syrup. He did

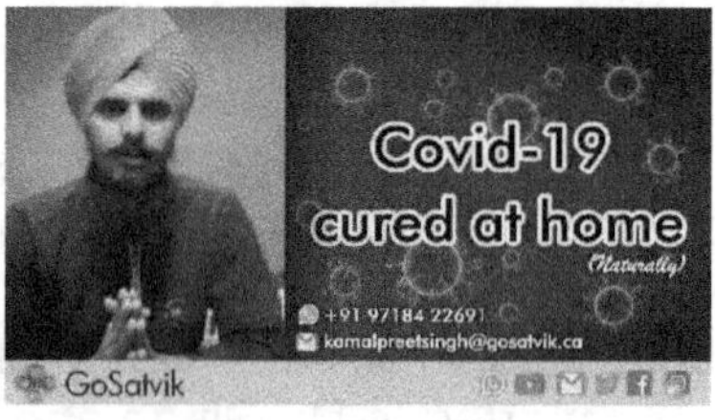

not get much relief. He reported to Dr. Singh and followed the 72-hour liquid diet protocol. He got normal in 5 days and recovered from all symptoms.

7. Manoj Mishra from Faridabad tested positive for Covid-19 on 17th September 2020 along with his wife, daughter, and father. He felt the need to be hospitalized. He consumed lots of drugs including coronil, vitamin-c,

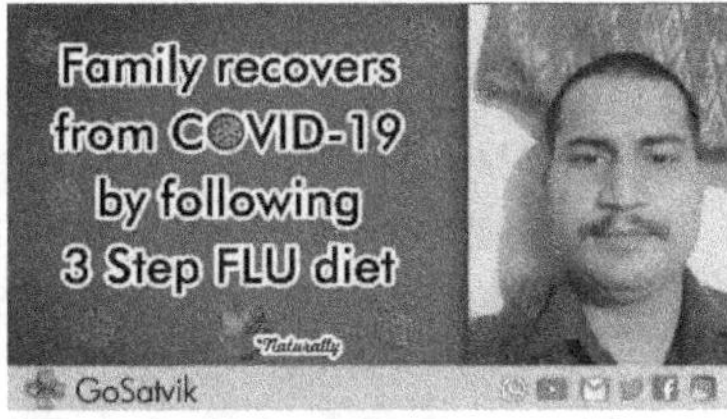

paracetamol, etc. But he did not get relief. He reported to Dr. Singh on the recommendation of his friend. He got cured in 3 days with 72-hour liquid diet protocol. He did not consume any drugs. All the family members tested negative for Covid-19 on 30th September 2020.

8. Sanjay Belapurkar along with his wife and son tested positive for Covid-19. They reported to Dr. Singh with symptoms like fever, headache, etc. His wife had a continuous fever for about 5 days. They followed 72-hour

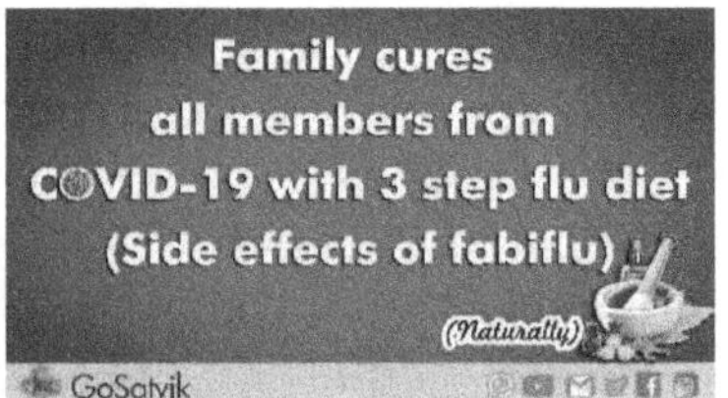

liquid diet protocol. However, they did not inform us that they were consuming the drugs prescribed by medical doctor. When his daughter told us that her mother is not getting better, we enquired about it. She said that she was taking favipiravir tablet as per the medical doctor's advice. We showed her the scientific evidence of the harm of such toxic drugs. She stopped the drug immediately and she did not get fever from the next day. All the family members got cured in 7 days on the diet protocol.

9. Amandeep Singh from New Delhi, age 27 yrs., reported to Dr. Singh with the symptoms of fever and weakness on 29th August 2020. He was tested positive for Covid-19. His weakness was gone within 24 hours of following

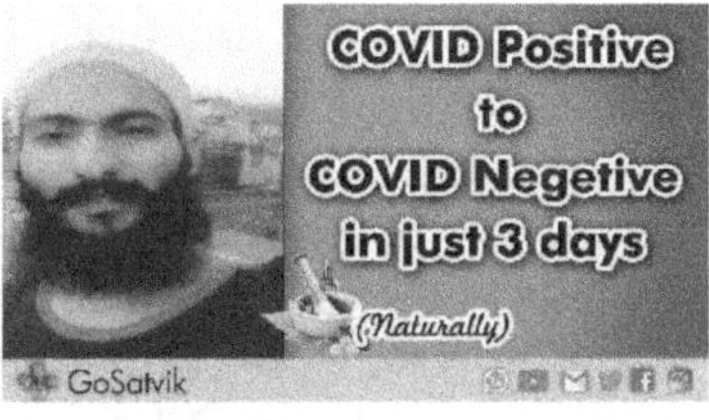

the protocol. He got cured in 3 days with 72-hour liquid diet protocol. He did not consume any drugs. He says it was the first time I recovered from an illness without any drug. He also tested negative for Covid-19.

10. Arvind Kedare from Hyderabad, age 40 yrs., reported to Dr. Singh with the symptoms of fever, headache, body ache, and weakness on 12th September 2020. He was tested positive for Covid-19.

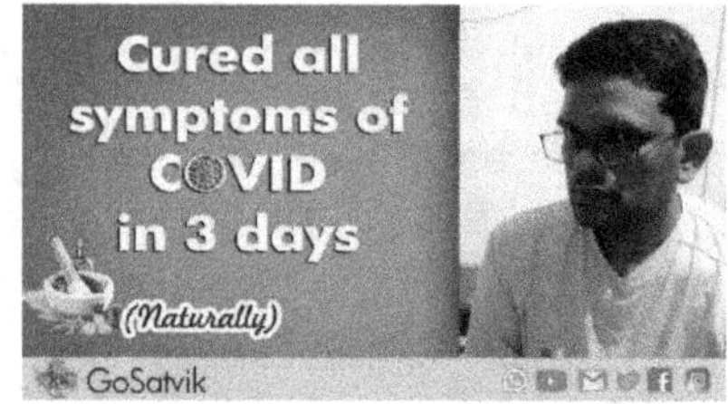

He got cured in 3 days with 72-hour liquid diet protocol. He did not consume any drugs.

11. Jasdeep Singh, age 30 yrs., tested positive for Covid-19 on 7th April 2021. He also had the medical condition of thyroid. He reported to Dr. Singh with the flu-like symptoms on the recommendation of his friend.

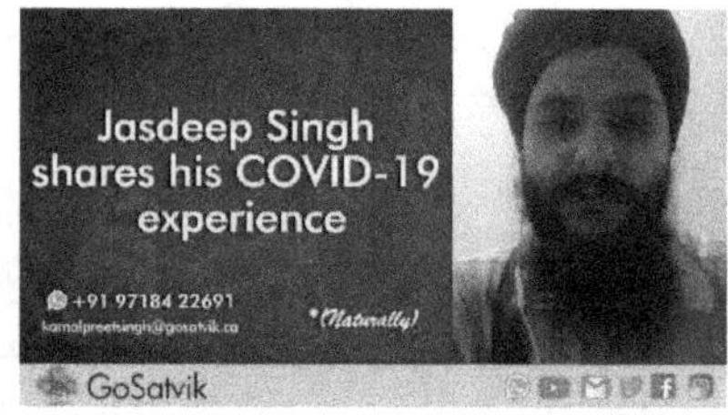

He got cured within 3 days with 72-hour liquid diet protocol and tested negative for Covid-19 on 13th April 2021.

12. Manoj Paramanik, a police officer, from West Bengal, age 47 yrs., tested positive for Covid-19 on 29th August 2020. He reported to Dr. Singh with symptoms of fever, headache, and body ache. He was also a

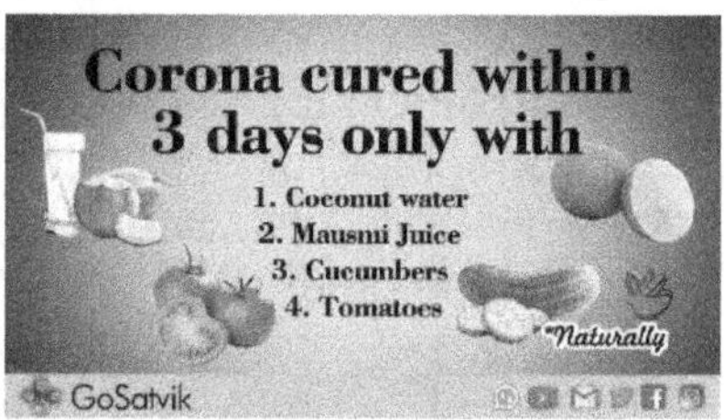

patient of type-2 diabetes. He followed the 72-hour liquid diet protocol and got fit and fine in 3 days. He says that he does not fear Covid-19 anymore.

13. Manpreet Kaur from New Delhi tested positive for Covid-19 along with her family. They had symptoms of fever, headache, and sore throat. They followed the 72-hour liquid diet protocol and got cured in 7 days. They

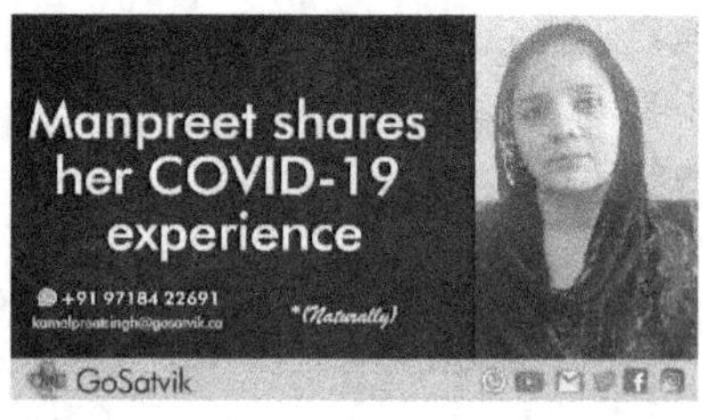

admit that drugs are harmful and natural healing is the best. She did not consume any drugs.

14. Ravi Patnaik from Andhra Pradesh, age 37 yrs., tested positive for Covid-19 and lost his sense of taste and smell. He reported to Dr. Singh and followed the 72-hour liquid diet protocol. Within 3 days he was fit and fine.

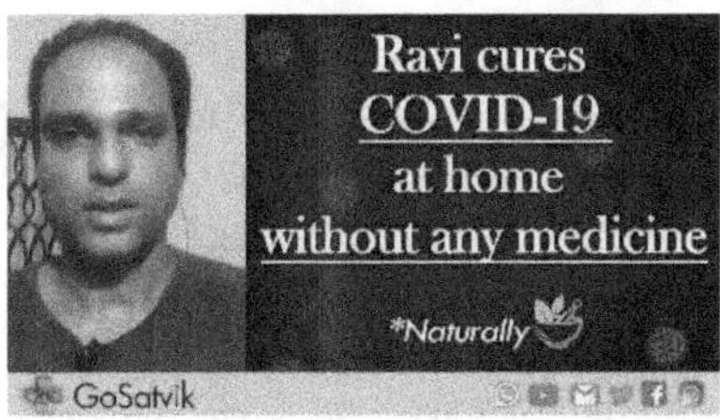

15. Jasmeet Kaur from New Delhi, reported about fever of her son aged 16 months to Dr. Singh. The temperature was 103°F. Dr. Singh advised them to be calm and do wet packs along with limited doses of fresh

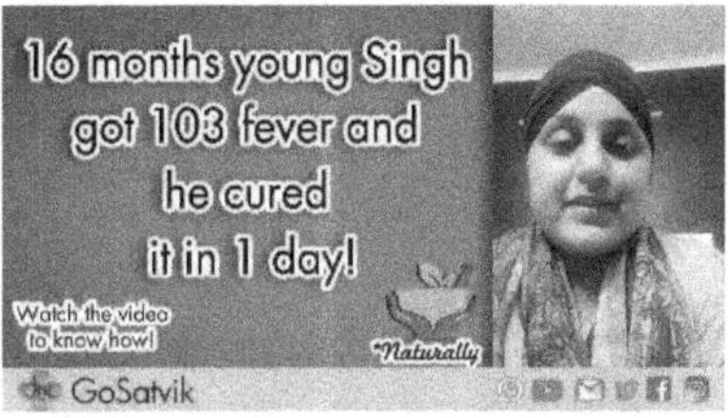

orange juice and coconut water as per need. His fever was down in 24 hours. They did not take any drugs. She also reported symptoms of loose motions, vomiting, stomach pain, etc. of her daughter. Dr. Singh advised her to do 24-hour coconut water fasting. She was recovered in 24 hours only. She did not take any drugs.

16. Harmanjeet Kaur from New Delhi, age 19 yrs., had fever, headache, and body ache. She reported to Dr. Singh and followed 72-hour liquid diet protocol. She recovered in only 4 days. She says natural diet and lifestyle is the best cure.

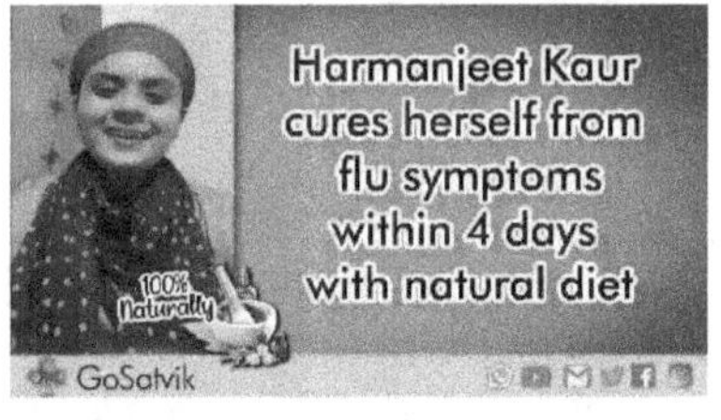

17. Jasdeep Kaur along with her mother and sister from New Delhi, reported to Dr. Singh with symptoms of fever and loss of smell and taste. She completely recovered from all symptoms in 1 week on 72-hour liquid diet protocol. She did not consume any drugs.

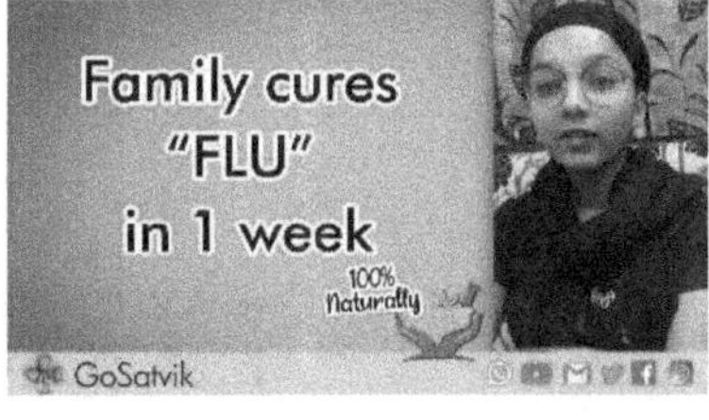

18. Jasmeet Singh from Jammu reported symptoms of flu along with his mother, son, and wife. His fever reached 105°F. He followed 72-hour liquid diet protocol under supervision of Dr. Singh. He got normal in 3 days without any drugs.

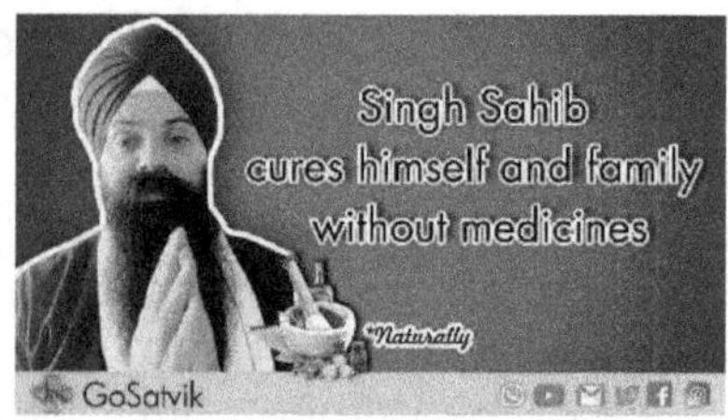

19. Ravinder Singh from Lucknow, age 23 yrs., reported to Dr. Singh with symptoms of fever, body pain, headache, cough and cold. He followed 72-hour liquid diet protocol and recovered in 2 days only.

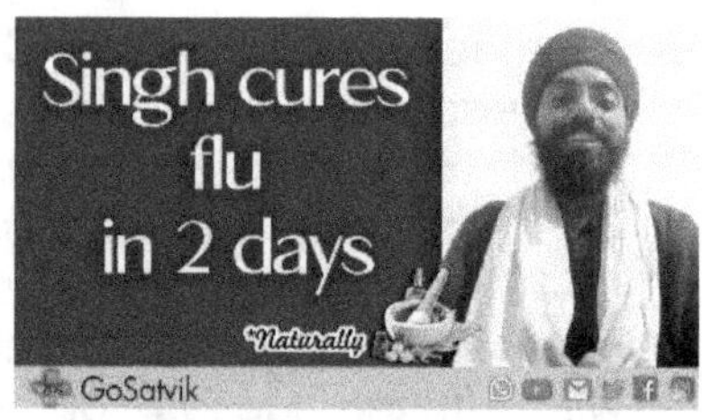

20. Suman Negi from Uttrakhand reported symptoms of fever, loss of smell and taste to Dr. Singh on 13th September 2020. She followed the 72-hour liquid diet protocol and recovered from fever and regained her smell and taste in 7 days.

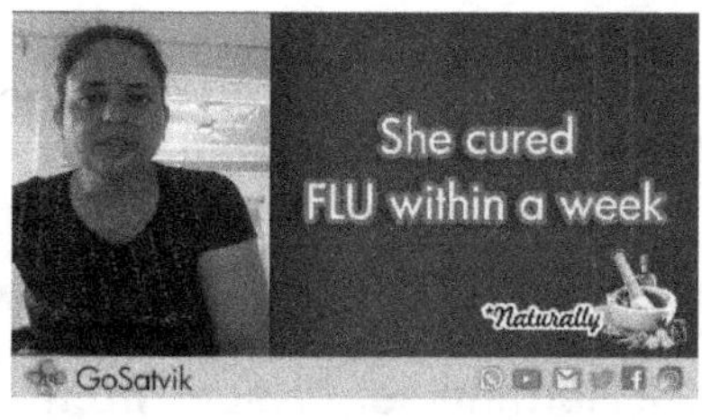

21. Sayeeda from Bangalore, age 7 yrs., reported to Dr. Singh with fever, and cough. She followed the 72-hour liquid diet protocol and recovered within 3 days. She did not consume any drugs.

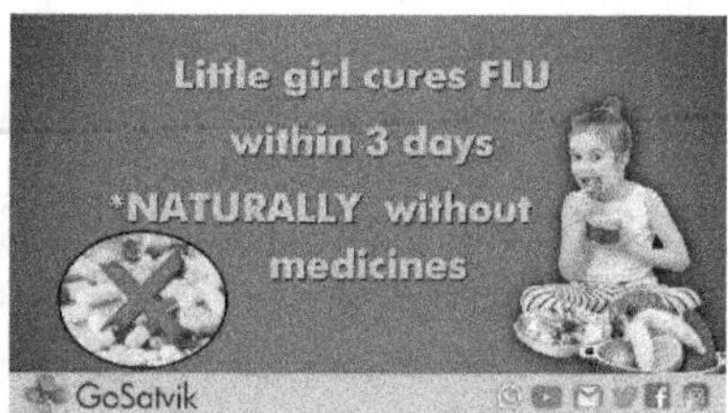

**You may watch their testimonial videos on
https://gosatvik.ca/mystory**

72-HOUR LIQUID DIET PROTOCOL

Day 1 (Liquid)

$$\frac{\text{Weight of patient (kg)}}{10}$$ (glasses of fresh Citrus fruit juice)

+

$$\frac{\text{Weight (kg)}}{10}$$ (glasses of coconut water)

Day 2 (Fluid)

$$\frac{\text{Weight}}{20}$$ (glasses of Citrus fruit juice)

+

$$\frac{\text{Weight}}{20}$$ (glasses of coconut water)

+

Weight x 5 (gm of Tomato + Cucumber)

Day 3 (Solid)

$$\frac{\text{Weight}}{30}$$ (glasses of Citrus fruit juice)

+

$$\frac{\text{Weight}}{30}$$ (glasses of coconut water) — **Breakfast**

Weight x 5 (gm of Tomato + Cucumber) — **Lunch**

Normal home cooked food — **Dinner**

ADVANCED NUTRITION THERAPY BOOK

Advanced Nutrition Therapy: Goodbye Drugs and Diseases is a Best-Selling book by Dr. Kamalpreet Singh that focuses on reversal of chronic illness through whole food plant-based diet. Delicious and easy to make recipes are provided to ensure healthy cooking habits. The book was rated in the top 5 books in Diabetes section by Amazon. Thousands of copies of the book have been sold within a few months of publishing. The book can be purchased from Amazon or through the website https://gosatvik.ca

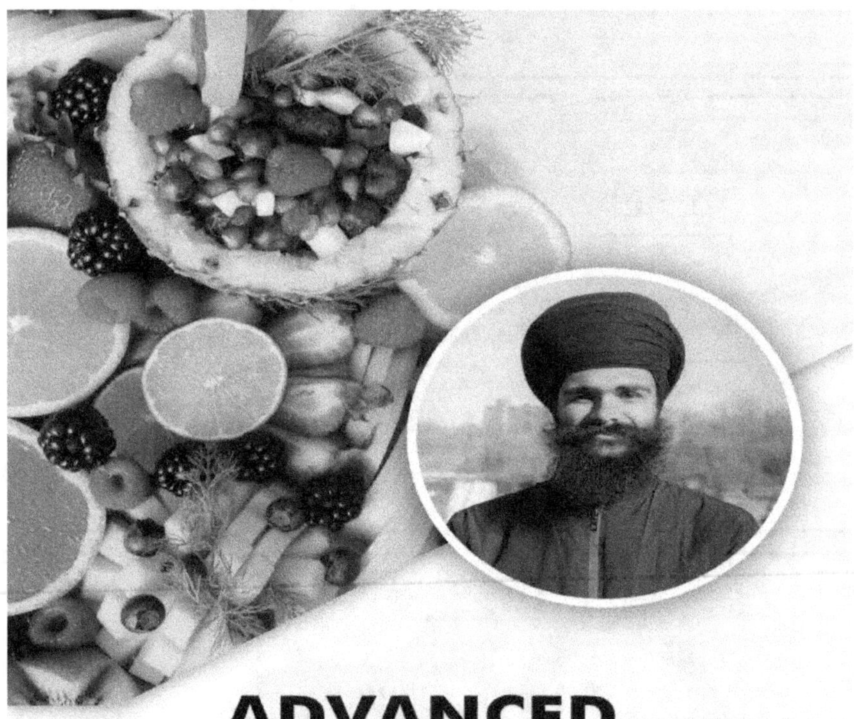

THE VACCINE CRIME REPORT

The Vaccine Crime Report gives you access to the findings of credible scientific studies published in prestigious medical journals that refute the claim that vaccines are safe and effective. The information in this book is extremely important for every person especially parents who wish to make an informed decision about their child's health. The book can be purchased from Amazon or through the website https://gosatvik.ca

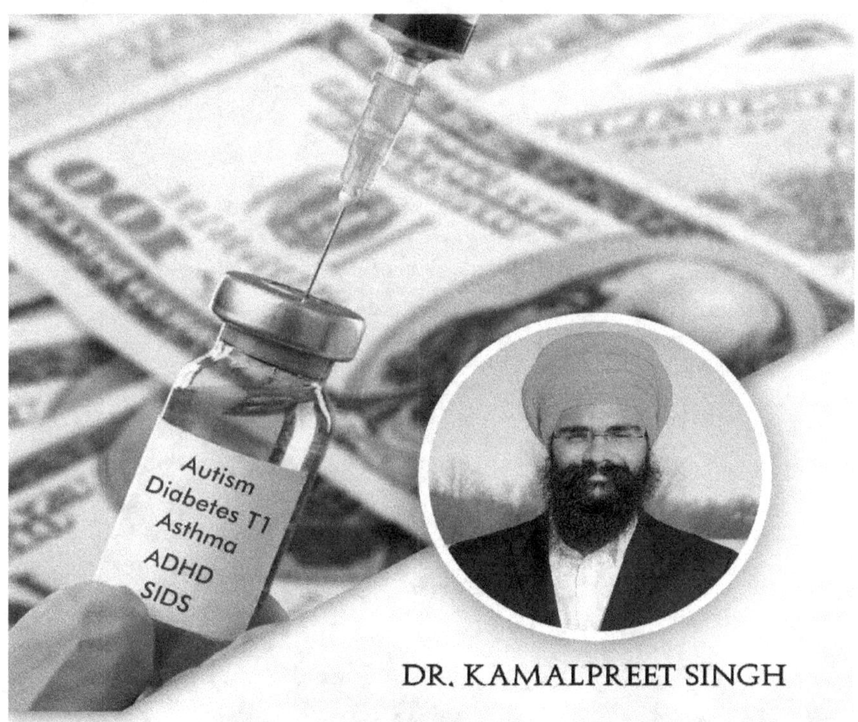

DO FACE MASKS REALLY WORK?

There is no scientific evidence that can conclude the benefits of wearing a face mask. At the same time, a plethora of evidence suggests that wearing face masks for longer duration can cause hypoxia, hypercapnia, headaches, breathing difficulties, cardiovascular implications and nervous system changes leading to exacerbation of existing chronic diseases, especially asthma, bronchitis, migraines, and Obstructive Pulmonary Disorder.

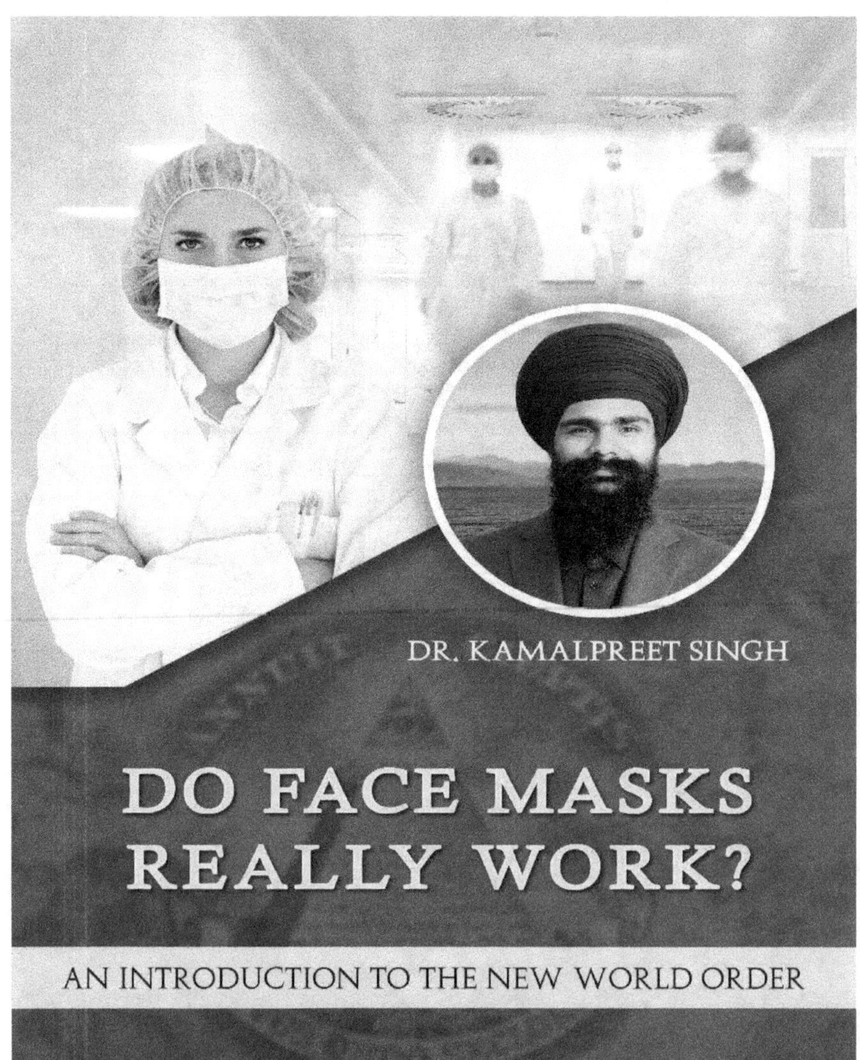

REFERENCES

1. S. Swaminathan "*Scientific Basis of Nature Cure*" Natural Lifestyle (2005), https://www.amazon.in/Scientific-Brahmleen-Acharya-Sheshadari-Swaninathan/dp/B08RCFRYD8

2. B.R. Chowdhury "*360° Postural Medicine – GRAD System*" (2021), https://biswaroop.com/360degree/

3. K. Singh "*Side Effects of Chemotherapy*" Go Satvik. https://gosatvik.ca/chemo/

4. K. Singh "*Advanced Nutrition Therapy: Goodbye Drugs and Diseases*" (2022), https://gosatvik.ca/books/

5. S. Swaminathan "*Science of Natural Hygiene*" (2005), https://www.amazon.in/Science-Natural-Hygiene-Sheshadri-Swaminathan/dp/B08CS3KSTY

6. A. R. Torres "*Is fever suppression involved in the etiology of autism and neurodevelopmental disorders?*" BMC Pediatrics (2003), https://www.ncbi.nlm.nih.gov/pmc/articles/PMC194752/

7. A. S. El-Radhi "*Fever management: Evidence vs current practice*" World Journal of Clinical Pediatrics (2012), https://www.ncbi.nlm.nih.gov/pmc/articles/PMC4145646/

8. J. E. Sullivan "*Fever and antipyretic use in children*" Pediatrics (2011), https://pubmed.ncbi.nlm.nih.gov/21357332/

9. P. Lagerløv "*Childhood illnesses and the use of paracetamol (acetaminophen): a qualitative study of parents' management of common childhood illnesses*" Family Practise (2003), https://pubmed.ncbi.nlm.nih.gov/14701898/

10. B. D. Schmitt "*Fever phobia: misconceptions of parents about fevers*" American Journal of Diseases of Children (1980), https://pubmed.ncbi.nlm.nih.gov/7352443/

11. C. E. Mayoral "*Alternating antipyretics: is this an alternative?*" Pediatrics (2000), https://pubmed.ncbi.nlm.nih.gov/10790455 /

12. E. Osawa "*Studies Relating to the Serum Resistance of Certain Gram-Negative Bacteria*" The Journal of Experimental Medicine (1964), https://pubmed.ncbi.nlm.nih.gov/14115824/

13. A. Lwoff "*Factors influencing the evolution of viral diseases at the cellular level and in the organism*" Bacteriological Reviews (1959), https://pubmed.ncbi.nlm.nih.gov/14419105/

14. C. A. Dinarello "*Mechanisms of fever induced by recombinant human interferon*" The Journal of Clinical Investigation (1984), https://pubmed.ncbi.nlm.nih.gov/6590569/

15. A. S. El-Radhi "*Association of high fever and short bacterial excretion after salmonellosis*" Archives of Disease in Childhood (1992), https://pubmed.ncbi.nlm.nih.gov/1580689/

16. A. S. El-Radhi "*Infection in neonatal hypothermia*" Archives of Disease in Childhood (1983), https://pubmed.ncbi.nlm.nih.gov/6338837/

17. A. Yerushalmi "*Treatment of infectious coryza and persistent allergic rhinitis with thermotherapy*" C R Seances Acad Sci D (1980), https://pubmed.ncbi.nlm.nih.gov/6784948/

18. N. M. Graham "*Adverse effects of aspirin, acetaminophen, and ibuprofen on immune function, viral shedding, and clinical status in rhinovirus-infected volunteers*" The Journal of Infectious Diseases (1990), https://pubmed.ncbi.nlm.nih.gov/2172402/

19. L. K. Williams "*The relationship between early fever and allergic sensitization at age 6 to 7 years*" The Journal of Allergy and Clinical Immunology (2004), https://pubmed.ncbi.nlm.nih.gov/14767444/

20. L. K. Vaughn "*Antipyresis: its effect on mortality rate of bacterially infected rabbits*" Brain Research Bulletin (1980), https://pubmed.ncbi.nlm.nih.gov/7363103/

21. R. H. Husseini "*Elevation of nasal viral levels by suppression of fever in ferrets infected with influenza viruses of differing virulence*" The Journal of Infectious Diseases (1982), https://pubmed.ncbi.nlm.nih.gov/7069233/

22. M. J. Kluger "*Fever: role of pyrogens and cryogens*" Physiological Reviews (1991), https://pubmed.ncbi.nlm.nih.gov/1986393/

23. H. D. Jampel "*Fever and immunoregulation. III. Hyperthermia augments the primary in vitro humoral immune response*" The Journal of Experimental Medicine (1983), https://pubmed.ncbi.nlm.nih.gov/6220108/

24. N. J. Roberts Jr. "*Hyperthermia and human leukocyte functions: effects on response of lymphocytes to mitogen and antigen and bactericidal capacity of monocytes and neutrophils*" Infection and Immunity (1977), https://pubmed.ncbi.nlm.nih.gov/412788/

25. R. E. Bryant "*Factors affecting mortality of gram-negative rod bacteremia*" Archives of Internal Medicine (1971), https://pubmed.ncbi.nlm.nih.gov/4923385/

26. P. A. Mackowiak "*Polymicrobial sepsis: an analysis of 184 cases using log linear models*" The American Journal of Medical Sciences (1980), https://pubmed.ncbi.nlm.nih.gov/7435520/

27. Z. Rumbus "Fever Is Associated with Reduced, Hypothermia with Increased Mortality in Septic Patients: A Meta-Analysis of Clinical Trials" PLoS One (2017), https://www.ncbi.nlm.nih.gov/pmc/articles/PMC5230786

28. N. Osterweil "*Acetaminophen Is Leading Cause of Acute Liver Failure*" MedPage Today (2005), https://www.medpagetoday.com/psychiatry/depression/2233

29. K. Brune "*Acetaminophen/paracetamol: A history of errors, failures and false decisions*" European Journal of Pain (2014), https://pubmed.ncbi.nlm.nih.gov/25429980/

30. C. I. Schulman "*The effect of antipyretic therapy upon outcomes in critically ill patients: a randomized, prospective study*" Surgical Infections (2005), https://pubmed.ncbi.nlm.nih.gov/16433601/

31. S. Eyers "*The effect on mortality of antipyretics in the treatment of influenza infection: systematic review and meta-analysis*" Journal of the Royal Society of Medicine (2010), https://pubmed.ncbi.nlm.nih.gov/20929891/

32. T. F. Doran "*Acetaminophen: More harm than good for chickenpox?*" The Journal of Pediatrics (1989), https://pubmed.ncbi.nlm.nih.gov/2656959/

33. T. Sugimura "*Risks of antipyretics in young children with fever due to infectious disease*" Acta Paediatrica Japonica (1994), https://pubmed.ncbi.nlm.nih.gov/7941999/

34. V. Vasikasin "*Effect of standard dose paracetamol versus placebo as antipyretic therapy on liver injury in adult dengue infection: a multicentre randomised controlled trial*" The Lancet Global Health (2019), https://pubmed.ncbi.nlm.nih.gov/31000133/

35. J. Cendejas-Hernandez "*Paracetamol (acetaminophen) use in infants and children was never shown to be safe for neurodevelopment: a systematic review with citation tracking*" European Journal of Pediatrics (2022), https://pubmed.ncbi.nlm.nih.gov/35175416/

36. M. Meremikwu "*Paracetamol for treating fever in children*" The Cochrane Database of Systematic Reviews (2002), https://pubmed.ncbi.nlm.nih.gov/12076499/

37. P. Nourjah "*Estimates of acetaminophen (Paracetamol)-associated overdoses in the United States*" Pharmacoepidemiology and Drug Study (2006), https://pubmed.ncbi.nlm.nih.gov/16294364/

38. A. S. El-Radhi "*Do antipyretics prevent febrile convulsions?*" Archives of Diseases in Childhood (2003), https://pubmed.ncbi.nlm.nih.gov/12818921/

39. J. T. McBride "*The association of acetaminophen and asthma prevalence and severity*" Pediatrics (2011), https://pubmed.ncbi.nlm.nih.gov/22065272/

40. D. Kristensen "*Intrauterine exposure to mild analgesics is a risk factor for development of male reproductive disorders in human and rat.*" Human Reproduction (2010), https://academic.oup.com/humrep/article/26/1/235/710117

41. A. A. Adjei "*Interindividual variability in acetaminophen sulfation by human fetal liver: implications for pharmacogenetic investigations of drug-induced birth defects*" Birth Defects Research (2008), https://pubmed.ncbi.nlm.nih.gov/18232020/

42. R. B. Walter "*Long-term use of acetaminophen, aspirin, and other nonsteroidal anti-inflammatory drugs and risk of hematologic malignancies: results from the prospective Vitamins and Lifestyle (VITAL) study*" Journal of Clinical Oncology (2011), https://pubmed.ncbi.nlm.nih.gov/21555699/

43. R. B. Newson "*Paracetamol sales and atopic disease in children and adults: an ecological analysis*" The European Respiratory Journal (2000), https://pubmed.ncbi.nlm.nih.gov/11153577/

44. I. Eneli "*Acetaminophen and the risk of asthma: the epidemiologic and pathophysiologic evidence*" Chest (2005), https://pubmed.ncbi.nlm.nih.gov/15706003/

45. W. Shaw "*Evidence that Increased Acetaminophen use in Genetically Vulnerable Children Appears to be a Major Cause of the Epidemics of Autism, Attention Deficit with Hyperactivity, and Asthma*"; The Great Plains Laboratory (2015), https://www.greatplainslaboratory.com/articles-1/2015/11/13/evidence-that-increased-acetaminophen-use-in-genetically-vulnerable-children-appears-to-be-a-major-cause-of-the-epidemics-of-autism-attention-deficit-with-hyperactivity-and-asthma

46. S. T. Schultz "*Similarities in features of autism and asthma and a possible link to acetaminophen use*" Medical Hypothesis (2010), https://pubmed.ncbi.nlm.nih.gov/19748189/

47. W. Parker *"The role of oxidative stress, inflammation, and acetaminophen exposure from birth to early childhood in the induction of autism"* Journal of International Medical Research (2017), https://www.ncbi.nlm.nih.gov/pubmed/28415925

48. A. S. Saeedan *"Effect of early natal supplementation of paracetamol on attenuation of exotoxin/endotoxin induced pyrexia and precipitation of autistic like features in albino rats"* Inflammopharmacolog (2018), https://pubmed.ncbi.nlm.nih.gov/29327281/

49. S. T. Schultz *"Can autism be triggered by acetaminophen activation of the endocannabinoid system?"* Journal Acta Neurobiologiae Experimentalis (2010), https://pubmed.ncbi.nlm.nih.gov/20628445/

50. S. T. Schultz *"Acetaminophen (paracetamol) use, measles-mumps-rubella vaccination, and autistic disorder: the results of a parent survey"* Autism (2008), https://pubmed.ncbi.nlm.nih.gov/18445737/

51. S. Jain *"The Food Book"* Satvic Movement, https://satvicmovement.org/

52. T. S. Cowan *"The Contagion Myth: Why Viruses (including "Coronavirus") Are Not the Cause of Disease"* (2020), https://www.goodreads.com/en/book/show/54786062-the-contagion-myth

53. K. Singh *"13 Proof that Corona Test is Fake"* Go Satvik, https://gosatvik.ca/faketest/

54. K. Singh *"The Vaccine Crime Report: Must Read Before You Decide to Vaccinate Your Children"* (2022), https://gosatvik.ca/books

55. *"VAERS COVID Vaccine Adverse Event Reports"*, https://openvaers.com/covid-data

56. K. Singh *"Truth of Face Masks"* Go Satvik, https://gosatvik.ca/masks/

57. H. Pourriyahi *"Loneliness: An Immunometabolic Syndrome"* International Journal of Environmental Research and Public Health (2021), https://www.ncbi.nlm.nih.gov/pmc/articles/PMC8618012/

58. *"Cumulative Analysis of Post-authorization Adverse Event Reports"* Pfizer (2021), https://phmpt.org/wp-content/uploads/2021/11/5.3.6-postmarketing-experience.pdf

59. B. R. Chowdhury *"NICE Way to Cure COVID-19"* (2020), https://biswaroop.com/nicebook

60. M. Barbateskovic "*Higher versus lower fraction of inspired oxygen or targets of arterial oxygenation for adults admitted to the intensive care unit*" Cochrane Database of Systematic Reviews (2019), https://www.cochranelibrary.com/cdsr/doi/10.1002/14651858.CD012631.pub2/full

61. C. Guérin "*Prone positioning in severe acute respiratory distress syndrome*" New England Journal of Medicine (2013), https://pubmed.ncbi.nlm.nih.gov/23688302/

62. A. Malhotra "*Prone ventilation for adult patients with acute respiratory distress syndrome*" Up to Date (2022), https://www.uptodate.com/contents/prone-ventilation-for-adult-patients-with-acute-respiratory-distress-syndrome

63. P. Petrone "*Prone ventilation as treatment of acute respiratory distress syndrome related to COVID-19*" European Journal of Trauma and Emergency Surgery (2020), https://www.ncbi.nlm.nih.gov/pmc/articles/PMC7670293/

64. J. Mancebo "*A multicenter trial of prolonged prone ventilation in severe acute respiratory distress syndrome*" American Journal of Respiratory and Critical Care Medicine (2006), https://pubmed.ncbi.nlm.nih.gov/16556697/

65. R. Obomsawin "*Disease decline before introduction of immunisation*", http://www.whale.to/vaccines/decline1.html

66. S. Humphries "*Vaccination*", http://drsuzanne.net/dr-suzanne-humphries-vaccines-vaccination/

67. P. Thomas "*Relative Incidence of Office Visits and Cumulative Rates of Billed Diagnoses Along the Axis of Vaccination*"; International Journal of Environmental Research and Public Health (2020), https://www.ar25.org/sites/default/files/ijerph-17-08674-v3.pdf

68. S. Rikin "*Assessment of temporally-related acute respiratory illness following influenza vaccination*" Vaccine (2018), https://www.ncbi.nlm.nih.gov/pubmed/?term=29525279

69. D. M. Skowronski "*Association between the 2008—09 seasonal influenza vaccine and pandemic HINI illness during Spring— summer 2009: four observational studies from Canada*" PLoS Medicine (2010), http://journals.plos.org/plosmedicine/article?id=10.1371/journal.pmed.1000258

70. B. J. Cowling "*Increased Risk of Non-influenza Respiratory Virus Infections Associated with Receipt of Inactivated Influenza Vaccine*" Clinical Infectious Diseases (2012), https://www.ncbi.nlm.nih.gov/pmc/articles/PMC3404712/

71. P. G. Szilagyi *"Influenza vaccine effectiveness among children 6 to 59 months of age during 2 influenza seasons: a case-cohort study"* Archives of Pediatrics and Adolescent Medicine (2008), https://www.ncbi.nlm.nih.gov/pubmed/?term=18838647

72. K. Rebelo *"Flu Vaccination May Triple Risk for Flu-Related Hospitalization in Children with Asthma"* American Thoracic Society International Conference (2009), https://www.medscape.com/viewarticle/703235

73. V. Demicheli *"Vaccines for preventing influenza in healthy adults"* The Cochrane Database of Systematic Reviews (2018), https://www.cochranelibrary.com/cdsr/doi/10.1002/14651858.CD001269.pub6/full

74. L. T. Kohn *"To Err Is Human; To Fail to Improve Is Unconscionable"* Institute of Medicine (1999), https://www.supersalud.gob.cl/observatorio/671/articles-14460_recurso_1.pdf

75. B. Starfield *"Is US Health Really the Best in the World"* Journal of the American Medical Association (2000), https://www.jhsph.edu/research/centers-and-institutes/johns-hopkins-primary-care-policy-center/Publications_PDFs/A154.pdf

76. G. Null *"Death by Medicine"* (2011), https://advancedmedicine.ca/wp-content/uploads/2013/09/How-Effective-is-Modern-Medicine.pdf

77. J. T. James *"A New Evidence-based Estimate of Patient Harms Associated with Hospital Care"*, Journal of Public Safety (2013), https://journals.lww.com/journalpatientsafety/Fulltext/2013/09000/A_New,_Evidence_based_Estimate_of_Patient_Harms.2.aspx

78. B. A. da Silva *"The alarming reality of medication error a patient case and review of Pennsylvania and National data"* Journal of Community Hospital Internal Medicine Perspectives (2016), https://www.ncbi.nlm.nih.gov/pmc/articles/PMC5016741/

79. K. Singh *"Healing Stories of Patients with Chronic Illness"* Go Satvik, https://gosatvik.ca/mystory/

80. K. Trudeau *"Natural Cures They Don't Want You To Know About"* (2006), https://www.amazon.ca/Natural-Cures-They-Dont-About/dp/0975599593